The Hospitalized Adolescent

Adele D. Hofmann, M.D.

Director, Adolescent Medical Unit, Department of Pediatrics, New York University Medical Center–Bellevue Hospital Center

Associate Professor of Clinical Pediatrics, New York University School of Medicine

R. D. Becker, Ph.D.

Chief, Neuropsychology Liaison Research and Diagnostic Unit, Department of Pediatrics and Child Care, Hadassah University Hospital, Jerusalem

Professor, Developmental Medicine and Behavioral Pediatrics, Hebrew University–Hadassah Medical School, Jerusalem

H. Paul Gabriel, M.D.

Director, Pediatric-Psychiatry Liaison Service, Bellevue Hospital Center

Associate Professor of Psychiatry, New York University School of Medicine

The Hospitalized Adolescent

a guide to managing the ill and injured youth

Adele D. Hofmann
R. D. Becker
H. Paul Gabriel

THE FREE PRESS
A Division of Macmillan Publishing Co., Inc.
NEW YORK

Collier Macmillan Publishers
LONDON

The Free Press
A Division of Macmillan Publishing Co., Inc.
866 Third Avenue, New York, N.Y. 10022

362.7
Hof

Collier Macmillan Canada, Ltd.

"The Amputation" by Helen Sorrells was first published in *Esquire Magazine* (January 1971) and is reprinted by permission of the author and the publisher.

Library of Congress Catalog Card Number: 76-1698

Printed in the United States of America

printing number

1 2 3 4 5 6 7 8 9 10

Library of Congress Cataloging in Publication Data

Hofmann, Adele D
    The hospitalized adolescent.

    Bibliography: p.
    Includes index. Foreword by Anna Freud.
    1. Youth--Hospital care. 2. Youth--Diseases--
Psychological aspects. 3. Adolescent psychology.
I. Becker, Robert D., joint author. II. Gabriel,
Hugh Paul   joint author. III. Title.
RJ243.H63   362.7'8'11   76-1698
ISBN 0-02-914790-5

To the adolescent patients of Bellevue Hospital and New York University Hospital, whose courage, fortitude, and resilient good spirits in the face of adversity have given us reward beyond measure.

The Amputation

More than he mourned for walking he grieved for the presence
of the leg, and more than for the dancing he hadn't, for all
his nineteen years, done much of yet. It became to him
like a lost lover, all things because all lost—the diamond
part of his self, fleshed like roses. He cried in the night
for its substance, and felt it there! there! there!
felt it itch, felt the complexity of its ankle, the satiny
socket; the authority of its heel; moved its toes and had to
touch the sudden stump in the darkest of darknesses
to know the truth.

Sometimes in dreams he had it back, the sunrise grass wet
and prickly under his bare feet. The leg was his friend,
his companion. He stitched it in place in dreams,
had it tattooed with his name. He balanced his big blonde
weight on it and spun like a dervish. The joy of that!

Waking, loss engulfed him. Waking again and again, grief
burned him thin and hard. The leg lay still in its grave
and he acknowledged the grave at last. He learned to walk
on a stubborn, bloodless copy of his severed limb.
And not to think about it anymore.

—**Helen Sorrells**

contents

foreword

by Anna Freud

Specialization in all matters which concern the welfare of human beings—medical, psychological, educational—has progressed steadily in our century, with each profession intent on deepening and widening its knowledge and on improving its techniques. It is only recently that this essentially positive advance has been challenged by a countermovement based on the insights that neither the human body nor the mind, neither the intellect nor the emotions, are separate entities which function independently of each other; that, on the contrary, they are linked by ties which if neglected endanger the individual. The schools were first to discover that there was more to their charges than an intellect ready to be taught, and that outside their realm there existed influences such as hunger, physical neglect, anxiety, conflict, which affect a child's learning. Next, the juvenile courts were faced with the realization that waywardness, delinquency, and criminality are connected with the absence of emotional attachments in the early years before the individual's social conscience is formed. After that, it was the hospitals' turn to be confronted with the facts that distress, bewilderment, and fear promote physical upsets and slow up healing processes, while, conversely, surgical, medical, and nursing procedures can exert lasting influences on the individual's mental state.

Understandably, doctors and nurses are reluctant to relinquish their concentration on the patient's body, with which they feel their skills have equipped them to deal, and to regard not the patient's illness but his whole person as the object of their concern. Nevertheless, starting out from the children's wards, a movement is undeniably on foot which aims at achieving just that. It may well be that the book before us marks a significant step in this direction, if in fact it will not lead to the final breaking down of the barriers between body and mind, as they have existed much too long in the eyes of the medical and nursing profession.

It is much to the credit of the book's authors that they have selected as the object of their study not the adult who—if not incapacitated by mental weaknesses—can, after all, cooperate with medical treatment, and can bring a mature intelligence to bear on physical upset. Nor have they chosen the young child in whom separation distress, irrationality, and bewilderment tend to obscure the impact of the physical event itself. Instead, they concentrate their efforts on the most difficult subject of all—on the adolescent whose handling at all times presents a serious embarrassment to his environment. Thus, they seek out a challenge which reveals all facets of the problem they have set out to solve.

They characterize, rightly, adolescence as a period when mind as well as body undergo changes which tax the individual's resources to the utmost. The shedding of infantile love-ties, the acceptance of sexual maturing, the assumption of social responsibilities are formidable tasks by themselves, causing serious upheavals. They become increasingly complicated if at a time when physical sensations are in any case suspect and upsetting, illness intervenes and the body, instead of being a potential symbol of pride, strength, and advance, becomes a source of pain, fear, deterioration, and shame. Illness in adolescence, as described by the authors, negates the very progression toward independent adult status which is the aim of this developmental stage. It threatens self-management of bodily functions, freedom from control by external authority; dashes hopes of winning athletic renown or attracting the other sex. No wonder that under these conditions the ill adolescent revolts—against medical or surgical interference which, to him, seems to aggravate matters, not relieve them; against nursing care which seems to return him to the infantile situation of having his body owned and handled by the adults; and against hospital rules which disregard his new need for self-determination. There exists, apparently, no easy way out of this impasse: it is either revolt or utter resignation, depression, and passivity.

The authors of the book accomplish the almost incredible feat of viewing the whole turmoil not from the hospital's, the doctors', or the nurses' side, but from that of the adolescent patients themselves. They are confident that this is the method to circumvent the worst troubles; to allay irrational anxieties; to eliminate unnecessary aggravations; and to create, even in the face of these stressful circumstances, an atmosphere of trust, cooperation, and joint endeavor.

Readers of the book are left in no doubt that the recommended changes of professional attitude and hospital management are the right ones. They can only hope that the authors will be offered the opportunity to put all their carefully thought-out plans into operation.

preface

Adolescence is unique in its process of growth and development. It is a period in the life cycle characterized by profound biological and psychosocial change. Not only is there the arrival of reproductive maturity and a rapid acceleration in skeletal growth, but these years also see the final steps in the evolution of a separate identity and in the acquisition of autonomy. These matters are clearly reflected in teen-agers' intense narcissistic preoccupations with biological integrity, heightened conflict over issues of independence, and major concerns about mastery and control. In consequence, illness and hospitalization in adolescence pose problems quite different from those experienced by children or adults. Effective management programs must be responsive to this fact.

Yet, prior to the past decade or so, hospitalized adolescents were rarely viewed in this light; nor were they often regarded as having unique needs of their own. Most of these patients were placed alongside adults on medical and surgical wards or, if prepubertal, were perhaps restricted to a far younger age group on the pediatric floor. Within these settings, teen-agers were expected to behave in that dependent manner characteristic of a child or to respond with an accepting and compliant rationality as might an adult. Either alternative is in error and wholly inconsistent with an adolescent's true developmental stage. To approach a young person with these expectancies in mind can result only in abetting his or her worst adaptational modes.

But in recent years matters have begun to change, and the special health care requirements of teen-agers who are ill are receiving increasing attention. Ever larger numbers of young people are being admitted to facilities devoted to their particular needs. And more and more hospitals are establishing some sort of provisions for adolescents. These may vary all the way from setting aside several rooms at the end of a pediatric or medical ward, as might be most appropriate for small community hospitals, to creation of large, separate units in major medical centers or institutions for highly specialized care.

There is, however, little direction or support for those taking this step; each professional is often left to find her or his way alone. Although the ambulatory needs of adolescents have been admirably dealt with both in numerous articles and in several excellent texts, and although a considerable body of literature exists on the in-patient management of children and adults, comparable information about hospitalized youth is scant indeed. In addition, few staff members have had the opportunity to gain special training or supervised experience in this field before embarking on such projects of their own. It is in remediation of this lack that we have written this book.

We have primarily addressed behavioral concerns because we believe this to be the area of greatest need. But it would be a mistake to consider that this is representative of the entire realm of adolescent medicine. This field is, in fact, much larger, including *all* the needs of this age group from the biological, emotional, and social view. Sometimes this discipline has been accused of overemphasizing psychosocial concerns to the neglect of biology. Such is, however, far from the case. Perhaps such misapprehensions have emerged because professionals versed in caring for teen-agers have been in greatest demand in contending with behavioral problems. For this is an area wherein others tend to feel most disarmed.

The goal of this book, then, is to promote understanding of the full scope of adolescent growth and development and the effects of illness, injury, and hospitalization thereon, encouraging the implementation of a health care system that will optimally promote the teen-ager's return to his normal business of growing up and realizing the full potential of his life. We have approached this task in three parts.

Part 1 is a theoretical examination of those developmental issues upon which our management techniques are based. This has been drawn from the classic psychiatric literature on adolescence in combination with relevant writings pertaining to illness in children and adults. Those few articles specifically devoted to this topic in adolescence have been given particularly careful consideration. Selected data on staff attitudes and interrelationships, both among themselves and between the patient and his family, were also reviewed in evolving the interdisciplinary or "team" approach. The most helpful of all these references are cited in our bibliography, offering further direction for readings and the expansion of knowledge beyond what can be given in the space of this book.

Part 2 offers a set of basic management principles applicable to all patients and begins by looking at the mechanics of organizing and staffing the ward itself. This is followed by a discussion of job roles and relationships and ways in which to implement the team approach. These matters are then applied in following the "average" adolescent patient through a "typical" hospital course and suggesting ways in which he or she may be given optimal support. This course begins at the moment of arrival on the ward; then moves through the initial history and physical examination, preparation for surgery or special procedures, and contending with the acute phase of the condition at hand; ascends back to convalescence; and concludes at the time of discharge.

Part 3 responds to a number of particularly difficult and thorny situations that inevitably crop up on every adolescent ward from time to time and pose singular stress to all concerned. These involve youngsters who act out behaviorally;

have devastating illnesses or injuries; are in the intensive care unit or require isolation; must face biologically disruptive surgery; or have special needs consequent to such matters as pregnancy, emotional disturbance, or mental retardation. We then look at those who must face certain death. A concluding chapter examines the legal and ethical dilemmas inherent in the issues of consent and confidentiality and minors' rights. These matters often pose difficult questions in caring for some young people under the age of 18. A set of specific recommendations on establishing hospital policies is offered.

We have endeavored to present our material in an interdisciplinary way and to make it relevant to the concerns of all professionals who are responsible for hospitalized adolescents in any capacity. Throughout, we have intentionally used the collective terms "ward staff" and "health professionals," except in those instances where the topic under discussion was clearly applicable to one discipline alone. In this sense we have attempted to write a book about ill and injured adolescents from a comprehensive point of view rather than to address the needs of any particular professional group. It is our contention that health care is at its most effective when delivered through a well-coordinated endeavor. While we view the contribution of every staff member as valuable in and of itself, each is still inextricably intertwined with the functions of all others. It is fruitless to examine the pieces without also considering how they interlock and combine to make a whole.

Thus we trust that this book will be of equal interest to all related professions and that nurses, social workers, occupational and recreational therapists, and ward teachers will find as much of relevance to their concerns as will physicians, psychiatrists, and psychologists. In addition, considerations of physical settings and staffing requirements together with discussions of the legal issues involved in minors' consent are also germane to the interests of hospital administrators and planners. The review of the dynamic basis of the impact of illness and injury and coping responses upon normal adolescence, as presented in part 1, should be of assistance to ambulatory care professionals as well.

But we must insert one note of pragmatic reality. This book does indeed present an idealized approach, and we are quite aware that its full and consistent attainment may be only incompletely realized at best. We ourselves have often been in violation of what we recommend. Major communications breakdowns, expressions of staff frustration or overidentification, failures in implementing the team planning conference concept, and the like have all occurred with some frequency on our wards, just as they invariably will on the wards of others. Ideals in health care are rarely fully achievable and to some degree are inevitably subject to compromise by the forces of staff shortages, overwork and fatigue, institutionalism, and simply by the path of least resistance. The implementation of our recommendations is indeed a constant upward climb against these equally constant downward gravitational pulls.

This does not, however, invalidate the presentation of an optimal goal toward which one can strive. Nor can we compromise our basic philosophy. We will always contend that ill adolescents are best managed through the application of firm technical and biologically oriented skills within a psychologically therapeutic milieu that responds to a teen-ager's developmental status and emotional needs. These matters are not mutually inconsistent; both perspectives are vital and integral aspects of the science and art of healing. We also suggest that the closer one can approximate an age-oriented response, the greater will be the rewards to the staff, as well as to the patients themselves. It is indeed meaningful to help a young person cope with the stress of his circumstances and successfully return to the processes of his own maturation. We also confess to the vicarious enjoyment of an adolescent's youthful vigor, idealism, and freshness of view on keeping our own minds open and our outlooks young.

We have come to our concepts from the accumulated experience of the past five years in establishing adolescent wards at Bellevue Hospital and New York University Hospital. Not only have we derived this view from a theoretically based understanding of adolescent behavior, but we have also come to develop our own observations and solutions from having encountered just about every problem, crisis, dilemma, and growing pain that could be imagined. We have grown from having no adolescent beds under our aegis to a stituation that sees a joint daily census of more than forty teen-aged patients and a thousand admissions per year. In addition, the primary care and community nature of Bellevue, in combination with the tertiary care referral system that predominates at University Hospital, has collectively provided us with a uniquely varied experience in meeting a wide range of medical and surgical problems in adolescents from many different cultural and economic groups.

Additional information has been drawn from some three hundred extended interviews carried out by A.D.H. with selected adolescents representative of a wide variety of conditions and associated circumstances. These were specifically designed to explore the patient's own perceptions about being hospitalized and to analyze both short- and long-range effects of illness or injury and coping techniques. Our illustrative case histories have been drawn substantially from this group. Although all cases have been changed in relatively minor ways to protect the patients' anonymity, the points they illustrate remain valid.

Our writing team was composed with a comprehensive perspective in mind. A.D.H. represented the field of adolescent medicine and R.D.B. and H.P.G. that of liaison psychiatry. A.D.H. and H.P.G. have worked closely together in establishing the adolescent wards at Bellevue and University Hospital. R.D.B., a former co-worker and valued colleague of A.D.H., joined to bring balance and perspective by interjecting an outside critical view. Dr. Leon Greenspan's kind assistance was sought in developing the important theme of managing orthopedically and neurologically handicapped youth. His vast experience in dealing with these problems at the Institute of Rehabilitative Medicine makes him uniquely qualified. Additional consultation was drawn from our nursing, social work, recreational, and educational colleagues to ensure that our recommendations were fully representative of the interdisciplinary approach that we espouse. We hope that we have presented the needs of adolescent patients from a holistic point of view with fairness and in a manner that will be of use to others.

In conclusion, we wish to give particular thanks to Alice Thielen, R.N., head nurse on the Young Adult Ward of University Hospital, for her special review of material relating to nursing functions; to Nicholas Lecakes and Nancy Beebe of the Children of Bellevue recreational staff for performing this same task in matters pertaining to their field; to Ilene Miner, M.S.W., Susan Woods, M.S.W., Annalise Zassoda, R.N., Patricia Ryan, R.N., and Rosalind Meyers, ward teacher, for contributing further to our knowledge by their daily example at Bellevue from which we have substantially drawn, and for proving that these methods can indeed be made to work. Our gratitude also goes to Rita Fox and Anna Bader for their tireless energy in typing the manuscript. No less can we omit recognition of the patience and fortitude of Charles Smith, Robert Wallace, and Claude Conyers of The Free Press. And last, our thanks to Dr. Anna Freud for her comments and thoughtful contribution.

A.D.H.
R.D.B.
H.P.G.

one

psychodynamic considerations

chapter one
Critical Issues of Normal Adolescence

Illness and the various circumstances that surround it represent a clear stress and perceived life threat for every patient. The ability of the individual to cope effectively with this event will be determined by the complex interplay between the nature of the disability itself, his or her own inner defensive resources, and the quality of the external supports provided by family, hospital staff, and friends. The resultant force of these vectors will have a crucial bearing on the patient's recovery and return to optimal function.

In this chapter we begin the process of formulating both a schematic knowledge base and a disciplined affective approach toward the youthful patient. We hope this will be helpful in rounding out and facilitating the comprehensive whole-patient care that has become the hallmark of adolescent medicine. For the most part we shall concentrate on behavioral, emotional, and attitudinal aspects and leave the description of organ system disease management to the respective subspecialists. Nonetheless, there must be the tacit understanding at all points in this book that we also regard the maintenance of biological integrity as an obviously essential matter of highest priority.

From this perspective the comprehensive management of the adolescent patient first requires an understanding of the dynamics of adolescence itself. Subsequent sections will integrate these normal processes into an age-oriented analysis of both the impact of illness and the nature of the hospital setting and its supports. This theoretical base will then be incorporated into a management approach for both the "average" patient and for those in less common but highly difficult special situations.

At all points, however, it will be important to keep in mind that the broad generalizations we offer are just that. Guidelines are precisely what the term implies and are not, *per se,* applicable to each of the infinite variations in human experience and potential. Appropriate modification into a carefully individualized plan for each patient is necessary. However, we do postulate that a firm knowledge of the dynamics involved, coupled with an exploration of the interaction between possible patient responses and general management techniques, will enable the development of a realistic approach.

THE ADOLESCENT PATIENT

The initial questions to be asked are what differentiates adolescents from other age groups and what is the rationale for proposing a special set of management techniques. In response, it must be accepted as axiomatic that adolescence represents a unique and definable period of time in the life cycle characterized by statural and reproductive maturation, emancipation, and self-definition. It is the final surge in the process of achieving adulthood, manifesting itself in a series of quite normal "crises" that bring inevitable conflict and stress to all concerned.

The advent of this process is heralded by the initiation of a sudden spurt in height and the appearance of the subtlest first signs of genital maturity. Major and profound physical and emotional changes rapidly follow. In general, the onset of biological changes precedes and sets the stage, so to speak, for psychological events by a year or two. One needs to be physically mature enough both in body-image perceptions and in the hormonal activation of instinctive drives to begin the psychic processes of emancipation and adult role definition.

To keep matters clear we shall use the term *puberty* to refer to those characteristic physical changes that usually begin somewhat in advance of the teen years. We shall reserve the term *adolescence* for the individuating psychological events starting around 12 or 13 years and signaled by the beginning of tentative movements away from the home. This latter process culminates some six to ten years later in the emergence of a mature and independent adult.

It is within this span that adolescent medicine functions. Historically, the growing awareness that this age group's health care needs are a unique fusion of biological, emotional, and social aspects began in the early 1950s. Increased national attention to young people gained further impetus from the youth movement of the mid-sixties. The concomitant widespread rise in alienation, youthful drug abuse, and changing sexual mores, with its attendant problems of venereal disease and out-of-wedlock pregnancy, have tended to catapult medical concern for young people into the foreground. In these respects adolescent medicine has come to be regarded by some as a sort of semipsychiatric specialty primarily responding to the urgencies of teen-aged developmental conflict and rebellion.

But to see this field in such limited terms is indeed in error. Although morbidity and mortality rates are lower during the teens than in other age decades, substantial disability does exist. Among inner-city youth in particular, surveys have confirmed an incidence of some 50 percent or more of remediable but often unmet medical conditions. From another perspective the rise in the referral hospital has resulted in the concentration of adolescents with a wide variety of major illnesses. Technological advances are currently preserving the lives of many children and youth who would formerly have died. Also notable is the increasing number of traumatic injuries, both accidental and secondary to violence. Thus there is now a significant population of handicapped and chronically ill adolescents who must come to terms with their very real limitations in order to achieve a measure of self-reliance and maturity.

Adolescent medicine, then, responds comprehensively to all these health care requirements, giving equal weight to biological, emotional, and social needs in an integrated and balanced manner.

PUBERTY

Puberty begins with the relatively simultaneous arrival of the earliest signs of an accelerated growth rate and incipient reproductive maturity as manifest in enlarging testes in males, breast buds in females, and downy pubic hair in both sexes. In the United States, the average age of onset of these events is 11¾ years for boys and 11¼ for girls; they are usually complete some two and a half to three years later (table 1). Thus, for most youngsters, rapid growth begins approximately one and a half to two years before characteristic adolescent emotional changes occur. Puberty reaches a peak at the earliest beginnings of self-definition and emancipation and is nearly finished in an adult-appearing body at about that point in time when psychological growth is at its most conflictual.

TABLE 1.   AVERAGE GROWTH-SPURT PARAMETERS
OF U.S. YOUTH, IN YEARS

	Height			
	Start	Peak	End	Duration
Boys	11¾	13¼	14½	2¾
Girls	10¼	11¾	12½	2¼

	Weight			
	Start	Peak	End	Duration
Boys	12¼	13¾	15	2¾
Girls	10¾	12¼	13¼	2½

Source: Department of Health, Education, and Welfare, *Height and Weight of Youths, 12–17 Years,* Vital Health Statistics, series 11, no. 124, DHEW publication no. 73-1606 (Washington: Government Printing Office, 1973).

Relatively less obvious changes in muscle mass and body hair in the male, fat deposition in the female, and cortical bone growth in both will, however, continue for several years more.

As set forth in the classic studies of Tanner, progression in the maturation of primary and secondary sexual characteristics closely parallels the rate of the growth spurt, with development of the former about half completed at the peak of the latter. The reader is referred to Tanner's *Growth at Adolescence* for a full discussion of these events.

It is important to note, however, that the average ages commonly used to define the parameters of puberty can be quite misleading, for the normal distribution curve encompassing plus or minus two standard deviations covers an exceptionally broad range. In girls, for example, pubescence need not be precocious if maturation begins between age 8 and 9, or necessarily be abnormally delayed if physiological immaturity persists at age 15. Adjusting this upward by the one-and-a-half-year physical lag in boys, we arrive at a possible range of normal pubertal onset for males from approximately 10 to 17 years. Thus at no other time in life is there such wide diversity in size, shape, and developmental status for any given chronological point in time. One need only look at the annual photograph of any seventh- or eighth-grade class to confirm this fact.

This marked variability in the timing of "normal" pubertal development has particular significance for our concerns. Quite obviously whether one is an early or late "bloomer" will result in a substantially different perception of one's body image than if one is average. In our experience, the adolescent with delayed development is likely to have considerable difficulty in securing a sense of self-esteem and may be inherently unsure of his biological integrity. Consequently, such a youth will be especially vulnerable to the threat that illness imposes upon an already compromised self-image.

The adolescent's insecurities are often further potentiated by our own responses. We tend to relate to others, at least initially, in terms of physical appearance. The clues that orient us as to a person's age and status and that in turn determine our own attitude and manner of approach are largely visual, resting in an assessment of such factors as height, weight, facial appearance, sexual maturation, hair length, clothing, and physical bearing. We do not confuse a "baby-faced," short, smooth-cheeked 11- or 12-year-old boy with a tall, muscular, sparsely bearded, 16-year-old youth whose eyes are level to our own. And we relate to them accordingly. Consider the frustrations that may arise in a young person at the upper or lower end of the normal range when there are marked discrepancies between chronological age and physical appearance. How hard it is for us to accord a 16-year-old who appears to be only 12 or 13 the full degree of independence, self-determination, and decision making to which he or she is entitled. To a substantial measure one finds such youths frequently responding to these external expectations—and possibly to inner bio-logical cues, or lack thereof, as well—by functioning at a more immature level than they might were puberty more advanced.

At the other end of the scale, a teen-ager who has initiated and completed his or her growth substantially earlier than the norm may often be expected to possess a comparable degree of emotional maturity that does not really exist. Particular problems may arise when unrealistic anticipations of an adult type of insightful and stoic accommodation to illness or injury fail to be realized in a 14-year-old who appears to be 18 years or more. Such visually determined misperceptions generally do not take into proper account the true level of emotional maturation. Consequently, the young person may be blocked from effectively coping with stress by others' intolerance of seemingly inappropriately immature behavior that is, nonetheless, quite appropriate for his age.

Another aspect of puberty that has relevance to our concerns rests in the gradually diminishing age of the initiation of these physical events and the lack of a parallel age drop in the arrival of formal thought and the cultural assignment of adulthood. In the span of only about seventy-five years the mean age of menarche has decreased from approximately 14½ to 12½ years of age, and the appearance of secondary sexual characteristics that would have been labeled precocious a few decades ago are now within the normal range. There has been a similar regression in the age at which other biological events occur in both sexes. The precise reason for such changes is unclear but probably relates to both genetic shifts and improved nutrition.

In contrast, although we have no parallel measurements, it does not appear that the age at which thought mechanisms begin to shift from the concrete to the abstract has similarly declined. Rather, it has probably remained relatively constant at somewhere between 12 and 13 years of age. As defined by Piaget, the capacity for abstract or formal thought is as essential to the processes of adolescence as is biological growth.

Certainly society's assignation of the ages at which youths may assume adult work and sex roles has not retrogressed at the same rate and to the same degree as has physical development. Indeed, the thrust for higher education and the consequent prolonged economic dependency upon parents has tended to extend adolescence for some cultural groups even further. Only within the past few years have we begun to see a confirmed shift in these matters, as exemplified by the reduction of the voting age from 21 to 18 years.

These discrepant directions tend to create a certain degree of contemporary confusion between a child's biological preparedness and his intellectual readiness for adolescence, which is further compounded by relatively unchanging cultural expectations. This cannot help but add further complexity to the psychic work load of the young person in emancipating himself and establishing his own identity.

One last point about puberty needs to be made. The problems some young-sters have in cognitively and proprioceptively keeping up with the rapidity of pubertal changes are not often acknowledged. Used to a slower and more grad-ual progress, they may be caught unawares by their sudden spurt in growth. An increase in height of four to five inches in a twelve-month period may well be disconcerting to a child used to two inches or less per year. Growth itself also proceeds, at least temporarily, in a different mode than before, with arms and legs initially lengthening more rapidly than the trunk. Not only are extremities proportionately longer but the body's center of gravity is substantially higher than before. Both events require significant readjustment in achieving postural balance and coordination. Some young teen-agers are indeed all arms and legs, and may be somewhat clumsy. Pejoratively crediting such transient difficulties to sloppiness, poor posture, daydreaming, or even minimal brain damage denies that these phenomena are the quite normal results of firm physical prin-ciples.

In summary, the events of puberty culminate in the arrival of full statural and reproductive maturity. For the first time in his life the youth becomes the physical equal or even superior of those who have nurtured and raised him and who have had inordinate powers over him in some measure simply because they were bigger. The implications of the assumption of an adult size and sex-ual function for promoting and stimulating emancipation and individuation are obvious. Other unique aspects of puberty that should be kept in mind are: first, the magnitude of the normal range in the timing of these events as well as the frequent discordance between appearance and true chronological age; second, the increasing disharmony and distance between the advent of physical growth, on the one hand, and social role on the other; and, last, the rapidity of the growth rate itself with the concomitant major shifts in body proportions.

ADOLESCENCE

As previously defined, we have designated the term *adolescence* to apply to that period of psychological growth when emancipation and individuation occur. These events are closely and inseparably tied to both the unconscious conflicts and impelling forces of adult sexual biology and to the growth of true abstract thinking. It is during this period that the youth defines and incorporates those characteristics that are "adult" and "mature" in the best sense. Thus the major issues of these years relate to the acquisition of autonomous function and the determination of one's own role apart and separate from that of a dependent family member. To accomplish this the youth must discover ways of putting distance between himself and those upon whom he has relied for nurturance, protection, and love, with the ultimate goal of taking over from them without precipitating their rejection and abandonment. At the same time he must explore and "try on" a wide range of possible roles in defining his ultimate personality. Resolution of the conflicts inherent in these processes are classically referred to by Erikson as the "tasks of adolescence" and the "identity crisis."

We do not seek to present a full analytic discussion of these tasks. They are available in the significant works of Blos, Erikson, Anna Freud, Piaget, and others. However, we do deem it of importance to define pragmatically the particular issues involved and their manifestations. This is critical to understanding the implications of illness and hospitalization in this age group. Any interruption in the youth's efforts to stabilize his emancipation or to define future roles represents a very real additional stress upon those inherent in the process of adolescence itself.

Emancipation.   As we noted, in order to become an independent adult, an adolescent must separate and free himself from his previously close and dependent ties to parents. Functionally, he strives to achieve autonomy and self-determination and to establish his own inner controls in regard to decision making, freedom of mobility, and social and sexual activities. The accomplishment of these goals is often executed through a painful series of inherently aggressive confrontations and testing of who's in control of what. In this, the youth and his family both seek to redefine their mutual relationships—to fix their relative positions in a previously uncharted sea.

Parents, who have firmly incorporated their child as an extension of themselves since conception, must in some measure now give up this part of their inner indentity and gradually relinquish control and supervision while still imposing appropriate limits on youthful experimentation and excesses. The adolescent who has grown up in the close warmth, comfort, and security of family love now experiences unexpected and confusing aggressive and impelling inner drives to leave this nurture and, in a truly unconscious sense, to take the place of his parents. On the other hand, neither side seeks to abandon each other totally but, rather, to find a new type of mutual adult caring wherein the youth has separated from yet looks to his former home for a sense of continuity and relatedness to the past.

Obviously, emancipation can be a matter of exquisite balance for all concerned, and it is perhaps impossible to complete the process without precipitating some degree of temporary and periodic frustration, rejection, and anger. Confrontation is the norm as adolescents gradually test and try out their newfound independence. Major struggles in accountability and control are classically epitomized in this exasperating exchange:

"Where have you been?"

"Out."

"What did you do?"

"Nothing."

But emancipation is also a process of erratic fits and starts. The adolescent may be close, confiding, and affectionate with parents at one moment and—seemingly without cause—secretive, distant, and hostile at the next. While indeed inconsistent, this is largely unconsciously determined and beyond the control of the youth himself. Thus his moodiness needs to be sympathetically tolerated. This is a confusing and sometimes lonely and threatening business as well as an exhilarating time as the adolescent attempts to come to terms with his own aggressive and sexual instincts and to explore the world about him.

For parents it can be an equally distressing time. First, they must endure substantial frustration in no longer being able to impose the same degree of control as before. Second, they must quietly and sympathetically tolerate the testing confrontations of their offspring while still providing affection and setting appropriate limits. Last, they must gradually relinquish a significant portion of their ties with their child who was and still is an extension of themselves, thus having to experience and work through a very real loss. But, in normal circumstances, emancipation inexorably proceeds to its essential end. And the now mature young person becomes the generation "in charge" so that he may, in turn, recapitulate the cyclic process of human existence in his own life.

It is clear that any protracted interruption of this emancipation process can be a singular problem for the adolescent and bears a firm potential for precipitating maladaptive behavior and even maturational arrest. The implications of the enforced dependency inherent in illness and hospitalization will be one of our major themes.

Role Definition.   The other major task of adolescence is the process of role definition. To achieve adulthood, the adolescent must not only become independent but must also determine who he is and, when it is time to move apart, must be able to stand alone in a comfortable and functional relationship with his environment. He must individuate himself intellectually, sexually, and operationally (functionally). In doing so, he will be able to use his mind creatively; to develop his own inner controls and moral code; to relate to the opposite sex in a mutually caring and sharing manner; and to establish a meaningful life style and work role within the community of his choice.

Intellectual development. Powers of abstract thought generally begin to develop in early adolescence, and the youth begins to explore a new capacity for ideas. He finds that he now has the ability to interpret observations, develop broad concepts, and discover new truths, all uniquely his own. Much as the very young child tactilely explores his body and his surroundings—in the process of discovery, definition, and even sensuous enjoyment—the young adolescent explores his intellectual abilities. Ideation in adolescence is often initially expressed in grandiose flights of imagination simply for their own sake and the pleasure of them.

These thoughts in turn are put in the service of idealistic creativity. Perhaps there is no more unfettered dreamer than the youth, no more perceptive, sensitive, and ungenerous critic of the foibles and weaknesses of the adult world. Youth is a time free of responsibilities other than to the self, when life has not yet been clouded by compromise or capitulation. The typical adolescent, in experimenting with a profusion of ideas to determine who he is in a holistic, universal sense, becomes highly interested in philosophical and ethical issues. He enjoys lengthy discussions in which he is stage center and may be particularly intrigued by spiritualism, mysticism, and meditational religions.

Intellectual abstractive skills are also often put to use as a weapon in the process of emancipation. The frequent verbal confrontations between family and youth wherein lengthy, involved counterarguments are posed against every parental position, view, and value are indeed familiar. Such counterattacks are an acceptable form of aggression in our society, albeit often exceedingly trying and at times even painful, for the arguments of youth are not only typically persistent but frequently perceptive, dead on target.

The multiple psychic services afforded by current concerns of youth about ecology are illustrative. Besides offering an opportunity to explore possible adult work roles, it allows idealistic intellectual experimentation with various inherent philosophical and ethical issues, provides for the definition of values in interpersonal relationships through expressing concerns about not polluting the other fellow's environment, challenges creativity in searching for possible solutions, and, by no means least, gives a chance for a real "putdown" of adults who regularly offend every conservation principle from littering to eutrophication. At another level, putting these thoughts into action, such as setting up programs for collecting and recycling refuse or converting trash-filled lots into neighborhood playgrounds, can be turned to use in the process of individuation and emancipation in the areas of mastery and control and constructive peer group interaction.

Thus, in a highly complex way, abstract intellectual exploration assists in the definition of who one is as an independent being in relation not only to one's family and friends but also, in more expansive terms, to one's place in the universe. It is essential to find meaning in being an autonomous individual so as not to become lost in the crowd.

The new intellectual strengths of youth have particular interest for us because the adolescent becomes quite able to perceive the present and future implications of illness or disability. He is no longer limited to comprehending matters in only relatively immediate and concrete terms. The adolescent is now capable of being an active participant in decisions related to his treatment and of assuming more self-responsibility than before. In many circumstances, he is sufficiently mature to give an informed consent and even to obtain health care on his own. No longer merely a passive recipient of the ministrations of others, he needs to participate in decisions made on his behalf in matters that were formerly the exclusive province of parents and hospital staff.

Sexual identity. Defining a sexual role has often been regarded as the paramount concern of the adolescent. Seen in perspective, it is but one of a number of preoccupations unique to this age. However, it is true that adolescent sexuality generates some of the most profound conflicts, not only within the youth himself, but also in relation to familial and cultural expectations.

To achieve identity in this area the young person must first contend with his rapidly changing physical state and new instinctive feelings. Intense interest in the developing body characteristically preoccupies the adolescent. Embarrassed pleasure at no longer being a "little boy" or "little girl" is often clouded by some trepidation over the implications of physical maturity. The search for a sense of self-esteem, highly vested in physical appearance, is a matter of primary concern. The measure of this rests on how successful one is in attracting opposites or, more simplistically, on how effective is one's "sex appeal."

Of course, not only does our society not permit the full realization of these drives at this time, but the youth himself—still unsure of his self-worth, incompletely defined, narcissistically oriented, and a product of our culture—is not yet ready to activate them wholly. The multiple forces of taboo, uncertainty, and fear of possible rejection all serve to deter genuine fulfillment in mature genital behavior. Thus sexual exploration, among younger adolescents at least, has a tentative quality even when it includes intercourse, and is often used exploitatively to serve some narcissistic need rather than to express mutual concern and sharing.

Because of these tensions, the youth's very real need for sexual experimentation is often diverted to other, more acceptable, and less anxiety-producing activities. Besides time-honored masturbation, a variety of alternatives may be involved. Fantasy, pornography, sports, music, dancing, and altered states of consciousness, both drug-induced and meditational, that give a sense of losing the self in time and space, provide such opportunities.

Obviously any physical threat to developing body-image concepts diminishes the youth's growing sense of self-esteem and sexual identity and thus bears a unique meaning in adolescence. Further, a disability need not be severe in reality to represent a serious crisis, but need merely be perceived as such. The processes of sexual identification are often far more based on fantasy than on fact.

Functional identity. The last component of role definition relates to how the young person will express himself as a functional adult. Critical issues here rest in such matters as securing an education, deciding on a career or vocation.

planning for marriage and family, and assumption of a life style, whether expressed in the form of the traditional suburban nuclear family or in a rural commune.

The process of defining an adult operational role is also inextricably intermixed with emancipation and the development of an autonomous intellectual and sexual identity. Thus we often see the adolescent most uncompromising in his plans for himself and often quite intolerant and derogatory toward the accomplishments of his parents.

On the other hand, the young teen-ager frequently looks to extraparental adults, both those he or she directly knows as well as those he adjudges to be heroes or heroines in folklore, literature, and in the public eye, as idealized role models whom he may seek to emulate. We wish to stress this point as being yet another aspect of significance to the health care of adolescents. For members of the hospital staff are frequently cast in such an idealized role. This may either be put to great use in supporting a youth in time of crisis or further confuse matters if the adolescent's unrealistic perceptions of perfection in a staff member are taken for anything more than the fantasies that they are.

The young idealist dreams of discovering great new truths, bringing peace to the world, eliminating poverty and disease, and winning the Nobel Prize. For all but a few, the abandonment of such idealistic prospects and the eventual, inevitable accommodation to reality signal the end of adolescence and the initiation of adulthood.

In concluding this section, we again wish to emphasize those aspects of adolescent development that may be particularly compromised by physical disability. A clear threat exists to body-image perceptions and self-esteem, to sexual identity concerns and attractiveness, and certainly to career and life style expectations. In general, intellectual functions will be impinged upon to a considerably lesser degree and may afford a very real strength on which to build.

STAGES OF ADOLESCENCE

It will be useful to extend the "tasks of adolescence" longitudinally, as young people are differentially vulnerable to the various stresses of illness and hospitalization depending on what point in development they arise. Generally, the young adolescent will be particularly threatened by conditions that influence appearance or limit mobility and the older youth may be most affected in matters that may alter career choice or marriage plans. Somewhat arbitrarily we shall divide development into three stages and look at early, middle, and late adolescence.

However, the boundaries of these stages are usually quite indistinct. Substantial rate differences in the progress of the various tasks also exist. Both caution against too rigid an application of these definitions. For example, a 17-

year-old youth may well be far enough along in emancipation to qualify as a late adolescent through a major commitment to a career and its educational demands, yet be considerably slower in his sexual role definition, still manifesting the narcissistic dating behavior characteristic of mid-adolescence.

We also wish to caution against the assignment of a specific chronology to these steps. While we do give approximate age ranges, these too are highly variable, colored not only by the youth's stage of pubertal advance but also by environmental and cultural influences. Therefore, we recommend that a teenager's developmental level be determined more by his current behavior and concerns as related to his particular culture than by age alone.

Early Adolescence.   This phase generally extends from 12 to 14 or 15 years of age in females and from 13 to 15 or 16 in males. At this time pubertal development is usually well advanced, and early adolescence can be considered to more or less coincide with the advent of menarche in girls and active spermatogenesis in boys. Estrogen, testosterone, and allied hormones are all at virtually adult levels.

It is quite understandable, then, that the young teen-ager tends to be dealing with body-image issues. He or she is eminently preoccupied with statural and sexual maturation and considerable narcissistic investment is placed in whether these events are or are not progressing at a "normal" rate. In our experience, many early adolescents feel that they are neither the height nor the weight they would like to be even when they are precisely at the mean in both measurements.

In addition, the youngster is also experiencing a host of new bodily sensations related to both increasing physical strength and prowess and mounting sexual drives. It is no surprise to physicians in adolescent medicine for many in this group to be intensely concerned about their physical status and to have a host of somatic complaints when they visit the office. It is part of the art of this discipline to differentiate those exaggerated minor physical discomforts that are a normal reflection of heightened bodily awareness from those that are neurotically determined or symptomatic of biological illness.

The major questions raised at this time firmly relate to these preoccupations and ask "How do I look and how do I feel?" This is expressed not only by long, solitary musings in front of the mirror, but also by frequent comparisons of the self to members of one's own sex, and forms the beginning impetus to the rise of the adolescent peer group. In these early stages the peer group also serves as another sort of mirror wherein the youth may examine his or her normalcy in terms of whether he or she seems to be accepted and liked or not. The most intense emotional relationships outside the home are with friends of the same gender, for there is a need to establish one's acceptability in this arena before being secure enough to explore relationships with opposites. In this

period, crushes on best friends represent the phase of normal adolescent homo-
sexuality.

Emancipation strivings also normally begin in early adolescence. The typical youth may spend increasingly longer hours away from home, but he or she
is generally quite willing to be accountable to parents and to accede to their
wishes. It is not a time that places inordinate strain upon parent-child relationships, and communications generally remain quite open.

If illness arrives during the early teens, the primary concerns and anxieties
of the youth are how this will affect his physical appearance, function, and mobility. As emancipation difficulties are not pronounced, the young adolescent is
usually not only quite willing to allow his parents to act on his behalf but is
also less overwhelmed by enforced dependency than he will be at a later time.

Mid-Adolescence.   This stage begins once the young person has achieved sufficient reassurance about his or her own intellectual and biological integrity
through comparison with peers of the same sex to begin to relate to the opposite sex. Ranging between approximately 14 to 17–18 years, when physical
growth is virtually complete, mid-adolescence is perhaps the most difficult time
for all concerned. Independence conflicts and efforts to establish a functional
sexual role are at their peak. This is the period that starts with group "dates"
and ends with "going steady." Still highly narcissistic, youths are mainly
preoccupied with how they are judged by the other sex in terms of both behavior and appearance. Their chief anxieties are whether they are capable of attracting opposites and whether they can adequately meet gender role expectations. These latter functions are now largely determined by the standards of the
peer group rather than those of parents. Not only is the peer group now the mirror of one's body image, but it is also the social monitor and behavioral arbiter,
forming a sort of stage before which members may try on and experiment with
various roles, testing their apparent success or failure.

Within the family the emancipation struggle is at its height, raising considerable tension and conflict on all sides over autonomy and self-determination.
At one and the same time the mid-adolescent must reject and rebel against
parental support and control in order to individuate himself while secretly
depending on them. For he is as yet unsure of the regard of others as well as
uncertain in his ability to control himself without external guidance. To fully
relinquish his childhood ties with parents before these issues have been satisfactorily resolved would, in a sense, leave the adolescent emotionally stranded.

The end of mid-adolescence arrives when the young person is relatively
secure in his sense of self-esteem, inner controls, and independence. He is now
able to move comfortably about on his own, manage most of his own affairs,
and make the majority of his own decisions. Heterosexual relationships are no
longer the relatively simple expression of narcissism that they were before but

are now in part beginning to be characterized by mutual caring, affection, and responsibility.

Illness or injury and hospitalization are tolerated least well by the mid-adolescent. For they pose very genuine threats to a number of normal developmental processes that are at a peak in these years. Not only does the youth at this stage encounter major difficulties in coping with matters that are perceived to interfere with the ability to attract others, but he will find it equally hard to adapt to barriers put in the way of emancipation drives. To be placed in a position of enforced dependency and deprived of the ability to master and control one's own life may in itself be nearly intolerable. When this is coupled with a condition that may in fact or fantasy alter the youth's feelings about his or her physical attractiveness, the resultant anxiety can be monumental indeed.

These issues must not be overlooked in managing this age group. It will be critical that the young patient share in decisions, plans, and prognostic implications as much as he realistically can in order to support constructively his natural drives for self-determination. Further, it is essential that the youth be provided as much reassurance as is honestly possible about the prospects for continued attractiveness in an effort to preserve body-image integrity and the sense of self-worth. To leave a youth alone at this time and to manage him only as a passive recipient of assorted procedures and treatments may well be disastrous.

Late Adolescence.   Once a heterosexual orientation has been established and autonomy fairly well secured, the youth enters the last phase of adolescence. Extending from approximately 17 to 22 years, this period is primarily concerned with defining and achieving functional role definition. In the forefront are such matters as education, job and career, marriage, children, community relationships, and life style. At this time the young person is generally making virtually all his own decisions and operating at a highly independent level. Family interrelationships have emerged from the stormy time of the preceding few years into a usually very pleasant and tranquil adult-adult type of relationship. Communications are again quite open. The youth will listen to parental advice but then make his own decision as to whether to accept it or not.

Much of his or her affective life is now invested in a single member of the opposite sex, although not necessarily the one who will be the ultimate choice in marriage. But, regardless of how permanent or temporary the boyfriend or girlfriend of the moment may be, the relationship is no longer essentially narcissistic but rather one of mutual sharing, concern, and affection. The importance of this dating partner in events relative to the life of the late adolescent now probably supersedes that of parents.

Illness and hospitalization for this nearly young adult has its greatest impact in the potential for blocking the realization of career and life-style goals and forcing alteration of vocational plans. Such can be well imagined in the instance of an 18-year-old college-bound youth suddenly faced with the prospects of blindness or the young apprentice construction worker who falls and sustains a resultant paraplegia.

CULTURAL MODIFIERS

Although we have defined the stages and tasks of adolescence in relatively precise terms, these norms can be substantially altered by cultural differences. For example, inner-city youth seem to mature emotionally on all fronts more quickly than others. Young people in this milieu tend to date earlier, become involved in sexual activity earlier, and look to being the head of a household sooner. In rural communities adolescents also assume an adult life style at an early age, although social and religious prohibitions on premarital sexual practices appear to be more effective. While we do not necessarily equate sexual activity with maturity, there may well be some discrepancy in the age that rural youths acquire functional role definition on the one hand and full sexual identity on the other. Upper-middle-class youths, however, tend to have a prolonged adolescence because of the emphasis and value placed upon a professional career and the persistent dependency occasioned by the many years of technical education required to achieve this.

Aside from these examples is a wide variety of other cultural modifiers that may arise from the ethnic group in question. One need only consider the unique situation encountered by Amish young people, Hasidic Jewish youth, or even first-generation Hispanic-American adolescents to understand that one can evaluate neither the timing or quality of normal adolescence nor expected social and gender roles without careful attention to the particular set of cultural values that surround it.

Other, more pervasive issues also affect the character of adolescence. One cannot ignore the effects of national political unrest. The profound disillusionment of normally idealistic youth caused by such devastating and demoralizing matters as the Vietnam war, the Watergate scandal, and an ever rising cost of living all have an incalculable impact on a young person's future adult role definition. This growing inability to have trust and confidence in the adult generation now running the country and the inability to find many worthy adult role models in positions of authority may have served to turn transient acts of normal adolescent experimentation and rebellion into confirmed, permanent new values. This may be seen in shifting sexual mores, dissatisfaction with traditional educational systems, and rejection of a complex, competitive, achieving, money-oriented social structure for simpler, more humanistic alternatives.

SUMMARY

In considering the needs of the adolescent patient a wide variety of factors must be taken into account. This includes the status of pubertal growth, the stage of adolescent development, and related critical issues deriving from both inner instinctive drives and external cultural expectations. Certainly, it is a highly complex matter to unravel the intricate fabric of individuation into its many components and their interactions. Nonetheless, this is necessary to understanding and meeting the patient's essential requirements. In its most simplistic terms, the prime concerns of the adolescent revolve around establishing an intact body image and sense of self-esteem, defining his intellectual, sexual, and functional identity, and achieving autonomy. Illness and hospitalization clearly pose profound threats to the successful progress of these events.

chapter two

The Impact of Illness

In chapter 1 we examined adolescent growth and development. We now turn to look at the impact of illness upon these years. But, before considering the significant factors of illness itself, it may be useful to review several critical developmental issues that have particular relevance here. These matters will be operative throughout subsequent discussions.

Heightened Bodily Concerns. Ill teen-agers are particularly fearful about what is happening to their bodies. Any insult that disrupts biological integrity is automatically perceived in a heightened and exaggerated manner. Hyperresponsive to pain and other abnormal sensations, adolescents often react in ways that seem to be quite out of proportion to what their biological condition warrants. But these feelings are age-appropriate, and very real. The levels of illness-engendered anxiety and perception of pain that are "normal" for this age group must be measured in terms of the adolescent's increased biological awareness and sensitivity to anatomical insults, not in terms of expectancies that would be appropriate for adults or children.

Cognitive Distortions. The emergence of abstract thinking and its application to role definition inevitably leads to a rich but also somewhat distorted fantasy life in teen years. Thus reality becomes easily twisted and misperceived. How a given disease appears to the observer often bears little similarity to how it appears to the adolescent in his mind's eye.

This has substantial significance in considering the success, or lack of it, of telling an adolescent about his illness and care requirements. For instance, Kaufman and Hersher (see bibliography) demonstrated that youthful diabetics have grossly inaccurate concepts about the nature of their disease even though subjected to a thorough instructional and educational program. It appears that adolescent patients conceptualize disease in terms of what it means in altering their body image and feelings about themselves rather than in terms of what they know academically, often perceiving biological deficiencies in primitive terms of punched-out holes created by missing internal anatomical segments. This is felt as a genuine loss of body substance that leads to a devaluation of the body image and a diminished sense of self-esteem.

The Body Beautiful.   In her or his intense involvement with physical attractiveness and normalcy, a large part of the passport to peer acceptance, the youth is naturally somewhat hypochondriacal. This becomes evident in an exaggerated concern about minor deviations from the absolute norm in biological development and about the wide variety of petty physical discomforts that the rest of us take for granted and generally ignore. Added to this is the frequent somatization of the intense psychological pressures of adolescence, also normally seen in these years. Thus, when these frequent feelings of something not being quite right combine with the reality of true illness, it is an easy matter to understand the serious implications for adolescent narcissism.

THE NATURE OF ILLNESS

The loss of bodily integrity and sense of personal devaluation consequent to illness raises both conscious and unconscious fears of no longer being loveable and of being abandoned. The ultimate expression rests in the fear of death. Such feelings form the deepest core of all illness-engendered anxiety. However, there are many factors in this crisis that substantially influence the exact nature of the patient's perceptions and responses. Such matters as age of onset, duration, prognosis, causality, interference with developmental drives, and so on all have relevance in determining the impact on the individual adolescent. We shall now examine these factors in some detail.

Autonomy and the Conflict of Illness.   Confinement and restraint are inherent components of illness, and the consequent limitations on freedom of movement imperil autonomy. Thus disability is particularly overwhelming to an adolescent who is ambivalently struggling for emancipation and self-determination. But matters are not always quite so clear-cut as they might seem. It seems reasonable to assume that no one wishes to be ill. Certainly this is a basic proposition of the practice of medicine. It is also true, however, that being ill sometimes has its own benefits and rewards. For all of us, society's expectation that we will be mature and independent at all times can be a burden. We all have secret wishes to abdicate from responsibility and return to the warm nurturing state of infantile dependency. This conflict most often occurs in the adolescent, who is at the peak of emancipation struggles. Thus illness may well be perceived at one and the same time both as a temptation to return to a state of being cared for and as an anathema to a burgeoning autonomy. Such ambivalence is always present to some extent in the implication of disease.

Age of Onset.   The age at which one becomes ill has a considerable bearing on its psychological impact. Indeed, there are specific times in the life cycle when one is particularly vulnerable to the stress of sickness and other times when one is better able to adapt. In general, illness and abnormalities that are congenital in nature or initiate early in infancy are much more successfully integrated into the personality than those that occur later on in life. Such defects have been a part of the self and dealt with as such from the earliest years. But when a condition arises at a later time it obviously becomes a much more difficult task to shift gears from developmental drives that depend on an intact body to ones that must now accommodate to biological deviancy.

This task becomes particularly difficult at times of normal maturational conflict. It has been often remarked that a child between approximately 3 and 6 years of age is singularly vulnerable on this count. Without question, adolescence, and mid-adolescence in particular, is also a psychologically devastating time for a major illness or disability to appear. It is especially difficult for an adolescent to adjust to physical handicaps. Disruptive therapeutic measures, prostheses, braces, and the like that would be well adapted to in earlier years may now be rejected as totally discordant with the youth's image of himself, even if this means giving up significant improvement in function. Even more, the young person's total inner drives are in direct antipathy to both the present and prospective limitations and personal implications of being sick. Here illness is superimposed upon a time of normative stress and may well be the proverbial straw that breaks the camel's back. From a practical point of view, mid-adolescence is, like early childhood, a time when elective surgery would advisedly be deferred unless the youth is well prepared and genuinely quite comfortable about it.

Chronicity.   Serious long-term illness and disability create a special set of problems for the adolescent. The afflicted youth must now cope with the limitations on function and mobility imposed by his condition as they impinge on his burgeoning efforts to achieve emancipation and autonomy. The magnitude of this conflict will depend on the age of onset of the condition, its duration, and the degree to which the patient has already integrated it into his life style. It will also obviously depend upon the extent to which the condition and its therapies have actually been disabling, discomforting, or visible and, in large measure, how this has been dealt with by the family.

Certainly long-standing, serious conditions will result in a quite well-defined and fixed set of emotional compromises by the time adolescence begins. This in turn complicates the developmental tasks of these years and the achievement of independence and role definition. Indeed, we believe that no matter how well a chronically ill or seriously handicapped youth has managed to cope with his situation he inevitably will suffer to some extent from varying degrees of psychological immaturity, social isolation, educational insufficiency, and vocational unpreparedness.

Moreover, old problems, heretofore more or less in abeyance, often rise to the surface and assume a new importance in adolescence. It is not uncommon for a teen-ager who has contended relatively effectively with a disability through much of his life to become reactively depressed or, alternatively, to act out in some way. For it is at this time that the youth comes to fully perceive the extent of the restrictions that will be imposed upon both his adolescence and his future hopes and life plans. That he must somehow respond to this new awareness of the true dimensions of his loss is most understandable. The severity and persistence of these reactions, however, and the degree to which they impede an ultimately successful adaptation in adulthood will be directly influenced by earlier childhood modes of coping. No less important will be the nature of the continuing supports he receives from those who care for and about him, be they parents, peers, or hospital staff.

In this context it should be recognized that chronic illness and its special care requirements have often been incorporated into the intrafamily structure and that in some measure the situation becomes egosyntonic for both the patient and his parents. First, the child or youth who receives special priority in the household because of his greater care needs often comes to use this manipulatively to secure privilege and parental attention. On their part, the parents may attempt to assuage their own ambivalent feelings of guilt or rejection through overprotectiveness and ever more devoted attentions. While this is just as true for the adolescent as for the younger child, parents may create an added problem for the former by promoting their ill teen-ager's dependency in order to block his drives for autonomy. This derives from their own inner fears of losing meaning and identity in their parental roles. It will thus be tempting for some parents to use the medical condition in such a way as to hold on to their emancipating offspring. Such preexisting patterns as these often make it difficult, if not impossible, to help a youth become autonomous even though his medical condition allows it.

A last factor of importance in assessing the impact of chronic illness is the social attitudes experienced by the afflicted youth in his community. Most people are discomfited and even threatened by physical deviancy in others and may find it difficult to relate positively to anyone who appears different or acts in an obviously abnormal manner. Children and adolescents are notoriously cruel on this count, often not only deliberately excluding their handicapped peer from activities but also teasing, taunting, and humiliating him. Such attitudes are also prevalent among adults but are usually less flagrantly expressed through simple avoidance.

CASE 1. A 17-year-old girl with Turner's syndrome, unremediated advanced scoliosis, and mild mental retardation (I.Q. 65) did indeed appear strange. The stigmata of a "fish mouth," neck webbing, and low hairline gave her a peculiar facies. The short stature inherent in this disorder combined with scoliosis produced an ugly, hunchbacked dwarf. Her retardation was quite evident in somewhat childish actions and limited verbal content. Long shunned by peers and adults alike, she sensitively spoke of the internal pain and confusion this provoked. It was bewildering and beyond her understanding that people on the street often obviously crossed to the other side to avoid passing close by her.

It is difficult to cite all the possibilities for functional limitations inherent in various chronic diseases, but clearly conditions such as severe asthma or compromised cardiovascular function may have their greatest effect in causing repeated and prolonged absences from school with consequent educational deprivation. The same is true for sensory and motor handicaps where there are inadequate facilities for special schooling. Conditions that distort appearance often impose their greatest liability on socialization, because of real or feared peer rejection. And situations that require considerable dependence on others for assistance with daily functions—such as using the toilet, bathing, putting on braces, dressing, and the like—may see their primary effect in blocking the achievement of independence and autonomy.

On the other side of the coin, the well-controlled diabetic or epileptic, the youth with well-compensated heart disease, or even the one afflicted by early Hodgkin's disease, with the very real prospect for a long-term survival under modern therapeutic regimens, should all be quite capable of a full adolescent experience. As such conditions require only taking medication and possibly following certain dietary restrictions, developmental progress should, in theory, be normal. Difficulties in adapting must be seen as deriving largely from inner distortions, misperceptions, and hidden fantasies and the unresolved fears of both the youth and his family, rather than from the impact of the disease itself.

Obviously, early, long-range, reality-based planning to provide the best possible developmental environment for a child or youth with a limiting handicap or chronic illness is essential. But too often this has been ignored, with health care during infancy and childhood geared primarily toward attempting to restore or preserve biological functions. And it is regrettable that only at adolescence and the approach of adulthood does awareness of all the previously neglected needs related to the development of autonomy suddenly burst upon the scene. Frequently this is too late.

CASE 2. An adolescent boy had had two episodes, at ages 10 and 12, of life-threatening rheumatic fever with carditis. On both occasions he was confined to bed for many months, first at hospital and convalescent facilities and then at home. Although residual heart damage was significant, he was medically quite able to attend school and to participate in all but the more strenuous activities. Nonetheless, no one had ever arranged for or insisted upon his return to school, or encouraged his ambulation. Each of the many doctors he saw in the clinic was primarily concerned about his cardiac status and, assuming somebody else had taken care of social needs, never spoke of them. His parents, deeply frightened by their son's near death and unguided by his physicians, hovered protectively and kept him in a semi-invalid state. Not until he was admitted at age 17 for an evaluation catheterization was it found that he had never returned to school and that he spent most of his days at home watching television. He was angry, hostile, depressed, and socially isolated, using the threat of his heart disease as a sword of Damocles over his parents' heads to get his own way in virtually everything. With very little inner motivation for change, prospects for this youth ever to achieve any real measure of functional adulthood were negligible.

CASE 3.   An 18-year-old Hungarian refugee girl presented a markedly disfiguring degree of thoracic kyphoscoliosis. The unrest in her native country had precluded early treatment when her condition had first been noted at age 12. She was not only grossly deformed by this lesion but also suffered from substantial impairment of pulmonary function. Nonetheless, emotionally she was doing exceedingly well. She had made some close friends, although she did little dating. But, most significantly, she had primarily compensated by placing her energies and seeking her identity through scholastic achievement and dealt with her very real physical limitations by preparing for a career as a librarian. Her attitude was bright, cheery, and optimistic. Perhaps the harsh requirements of independence and resourcefulness necessitated by escaping from her country, coupled with the clear love and support of her parents, combined to facilitate this result.

How and why two such diametrically opposite resolutions of chronic illness can occur is not always so clear as in these cases. Frequently the reasons are much more obscure. But in some measure the outcome inevitably depends upon the degree to which normal maturational pursuits are resumed after the initial insult. This in turn depends upon the encouragement and support of those surrounding the child or youth to proceed with his developmental tasks in as full a way as realistically possible. Underlying this, however, is the fundamental nature of the patient himself and whatever inner strengths and resources he can bring to bear.

The Course of Illness.   Not all chronic diseases are persistent and unchanging. When a previously stable state takes a downward turn, the primary perception of both the youth and his family often is that of impending death, even if a fatal outcome is not necessarily medically implicit. Thus many of the same responses experienced by the dying adolescent and his family are operative here as well (see chapter 12). When progressive debility does indeed result in increasing physical discomfort, further restriction in function, heightened dependency requirements, greater isolation from peer contacts, and more compromises with normal age pursuits, it can be difficult indeed to continue to maintain a hopeful outlook.

In many ways a variety of maladaptive responses are inevitable companions to deterioration. Until the condition stabilizes again and forward-looking goals can be reinstituted, this will be a time largely devoted to a primitive "holding on" and to simple efforts at survival. The patient will focus mainly on the illness itself, with either an intense preoccupation with every therapeutic detail or an equally intense denial. All the psychodynamic factors of object-loss and the concomitant methods of dealing with it from depression, avoidance, anger, panic, or acting out to the mourning process itself are inherent in a progressive downward course.

At the other end of the spectrum is the situation of the adolescent whose chronic disease has been substantially ameliorated and who is now in posses-sion of a more normally functioning body than the one he has coped with for many years. The problems posed by having to set up a new personality struc-ture that no longer need adapt to a restricting handicap can indeed be monumen-tal. Consider, for instance, a youth who has undergone corrective surgery for congenital heart disease or some other such disorder. The childhood incorpo-ration of the limits imposed by his cardiac abnormality are now part of the ado-lescent's life style. Even though the biological need for these adaptations no longer exists, distortions, confusion, and conflict about one's self-image not only persist but may even be exacerbated.

CASES 4 and 5.   Two 15-year-old Puerto Rican males had been born with urogenital abnormalities: one, hypospadias, and the other, epispadias and extrophy of the bladder. For both youths repair of their lesions had taken place intermittently over many years and in early childhood neither had voided normally. It was not until they were approximately 12 years old that plastic repairs of their penises were completed; the boy with hypospadias then urinated normally, and the youth with extrophy was subjected to a Bricker procedure. At age 15 they both had functional adult genitalia; both masturbated with erection, orgasm, and ejaculation; and one was sexually ac-tive. Despite the great improvement in their anatomical status and reproductive capacity, draw-a-figure tests indicated that they had persistent, serious body-image deficiencies and castration conflicts. Male figures were shrouded and handless, obs-cured in one by a gownlike cape and in the other by torrents of blood flowing like a waterfall from the neck. Female figures were clearly malevolent and sexually aggres-sive. It should be further noted that at no point prior to this hospitalization for their annual renal function evaluation had anyone, either parents or hospital staff, ever discussed their reproductive status with them or uncovered their intense concern and fears about their abnormalities. One of these boys responded to his former genital dysfunction by becoming a Don Juan. The other met his sexual confusions by with-drawing from all contact with the opposite sex and an overinvestment in athletic prowess.

Although medicine expects that all patients will joyously welcome restitu-tion, this may not always be so. A youth who has come to accept disease-related cautions and prohibitions as part of his inner self may retain these perceptions well beyond any need for doing so, either physically or psychologically. It is as if emotional adaptations to long-term disease become some of the building blocks in the structure of the personality. Pulling them out loosens all the others and threatens to cause all one's psychic defenses to come tumbling down.

CASE 6. An 18-year-old girl had first begun having recurrent acute episodes of epigastric pain at age 13, but it had been diagnosed as psychosomatic in origin. Not until five years later was the true diagnosis of cholelithiasis established. However, despite an uneventful cholecystectomy, her symptoms persisted and two months later she was reexplored, but no further pathology was found. Subsequently, she had no further abdominal pain, but a not unusual postoperative urinary retention persisted. She remained unable to void spontaneously during the ensuing five months and required an indwelling catheter. No organic cause for this was uncovered, but on psychiatric evaluation it was quite clear that the abdominal pain secondary to her cholelithiasis had become so incorporated into the processes of adolescent body-image definition that when this was removed some other, now hysterical, symptom had to be created to take its place. At a deeper level this entire mechanism had its origin in long-standing difficulty in her sexual role identification.

Another distortion in the prospect for rehabilitation may be the opposite of the preceding, an overinvestment in the outcome with flagrantly unreal expectations and dreams of glory. This may be illustrated by the hopes for full normalcy in a youth with severe cerebral palsy undergoing a single tendon transplant or the fantasies about the instant popularity that will result upon plastic correction of a deformed feature. Adolescents are particularly prone to idealizing these prospects, both because of their heightened fantasy life and because of their intense preoccupation with and desire for bodily normalcy and attractiveness.

To some degree medicine promotes adolescent fantasies. In their efforts to reassure an anxious patient and to promote acceptance of proposed therapies, doctors may well convey expectancies of a greater return of function or improved appearance than is realistic. In part, these distortions may also arise from the physician's own inner fantasies of omnipotence. These hidden messages will be easily sensed and picked up by the youth and turned to his own devices.

Obviously, the sum of all these forces may produce a set of idealistic prospects that can in no way be fulfilled. Disappointment, disillusionment, and even deep depression are not unusual when postoperative fact collides with preoperative fantasy.

Of course, we have painted matters related to restitution with a very broad brush. In the majority of instances these issues, modified in various degrees by realistic expectations, will be much less pervasive. Nevertheless, by stressing these possibilities we do hope to emphasize the essential need to deal openly, honestly, and pragmatically with the adolescent patient, helping him or her to function as a partner in care. It is thus that the most constructive acceptance can be fostered and unrealistic hopes diminished.

Interruption of Mastery and Control.   It is critical to the achievement of autonomy during the teen years for the young person to come to ever greater levels of mastery and control of himself and his environment. Thus the adolescent, and in particular the adolescent male, is highly vulnerable to medical conditions that interfere with such activities.

Although it appears that sex roles may well be shifting and that new cultural assignments as to what is meant by being "masculine" or "feminine" may be in the offing, to a large extent traditional gender role expectancies are still very much operative for most youngsters. Boys are still culturally programmed to become strong, masterful, and successful hunters. In preparation for this role, the young adolescent male who excels at competitive sports and demonstrates leadership qualities still secures the esteem not only of his peers but of adults as well. Witness the social phenomena of little league baseball. Such esteem is, as we have noted, a prerequisite for the furtherance of role definition and sexual identity. Where competitive sports may not be so culturally "in," acceptable masculine activities are nonetheless still nearly all action-oriented and invested in "doing"—in other words, in coming to master and control the environment. Consequently, conditions that block action-oriented successes, particularly in early and mid-adolescence, will be most stressful on males.

Girls, on the other hand, while by no means exempt from similar distresses, are often much less distraught by the physical restraints of illness, which are more consistent with the greater passivity and receptiveness inherent in female role function expectancies. In principle, one may object to such sex steryotyping, but in practice we have repeatedly found this to be true among adolescent patients from a wide variety of cultural subgroups. Of course, these responses are by no means rigidly sex-assigned. Girls as well as boys often display considerable anxiety occasioned by immobilization. It is simply more common among boys.

Thus the young, teen-aged male who faces amputation for an osteogenic sarcoma, or who must remain in a cast, brace, or traction for a prolonged period of time, or who is subject to restrictive treatments, such as weeks of intravenous therapy for osteomyelitis, may react to this stress in a highly maladaptive manner.

CASE 7.   A 13-year-old boy fractured his femur in a bicycling accident. Once placed in traction and stabilized, he was put in a side room where he received only routine ministrations by the ward staff. From his perspective he was tended to inadequately and there were unwarranted delays in responding to his calls for attention. He felt that he had been abandoned. But the more he complained, the more he gained a reputation as a troublemaker and the more the staff tended to avoid him. Becoming acutely depressed and withdrawn, he eventually made a suicidal gesture by attempting to hang himself in his traction cords.

Admittedly, the above case represents a highly unusual and exaggerated response. But it does point up the significant levels of anxiety and depression that may be occasioned by even not serious conditions. What is critical, here, is the immobilization and not the implications of the illness itself.

Responses to interference with mastery and control need not take the form of a depressive mode; numerous alternatives are available, as detailed in chapter 4. These may be either constructive—as are intellectualization and compensation—or maladaptive—as are acting out, panic, and persistant regression. But, regardless of just how the situation is coped with, members of the health care team should be particularly alert to the singular needs of the adolescent whose condition significantly limits activity and interferes with mastery and control.

Visibility.   Whether an illness interferes with the adolescent's perceptions of her or his attractiveness is also a critical issue of these years. Here the teenaged girl is particularly vulnerable, though the teen-aged boy is by no means unconcerned. Here too early and mid-adolescents are most susceptible. Fears of possible mutilation, loss of the ability to attract opposites, and ultimate abandonment are at the core.

CASES 8 and 9.   Two 16-year-olds, one male and one female, had long-standing, severe, and highly obvious psoriasis involving the face and extremities. The boy, active in sports and on the high school basketball team, was most concerned about the limiting demands of the prescribed two-hour daily self-treatment regimen. This seriously interfered with his athletics. His solution was to forget about treatment unless the attendant pruritus became unbearable. In addition he hospitalized himself several times a year for intensive therapy to keep the condition in check. He was not particularly bothered by his appearance and was emotionally quite comfortable in his revealing basketball uniform, even in public.

In contrast, the girl's main preoccupation was how she looked to others, even to the point of having some mildly paranoid ideation. Without fail she rigorously pursued her extensive treatment program each day, often limiting socialization in order to do so. In addition, her clothing and hair style were selected primarily to hide her lesions as much as possible.

Physical distortions, visible handicaps, scars, skin rashes, unsightly blemishes, and other such disfigurements often assume infinitely greater proportions in the adolescent's mind than do any other factors relating to the situation. Thus an adolescent girl with lupus erythematosus may be much more preoccupied with her malar rash than the condition itself. Or the youth with a brain tumor undergoing radiation therapy may be much more concerned about possible alopecia than about the implications of the underlying lesion. Certainly, the need of such teen-agers to hide the visible signs of their illness as much as is realistically possible must be recognized and supported if the very real potential for maladaptive withdrawal and isolation is to be avoided. At times, enhancing appearance may even need be at the expense of enhancing function. Teen-agers who require prostheses or braces, for example, are often much more interested in the physical appearance of these devices than in an improvement in their ability to get about.

On the other hand, nonvisible conditions bring their own special set of problems. Whereas obvious illnesses and handicaps can be measured and assessed in terms of a clear and visible reality, conditions not so readily apparent are much more difficult to assess and may provoke a far greater confusion in self-perception and body image. The adolescent's facility to come to such conclusions, due to his new ability for abstract thinking and rich fantasy life, lead to very real differences in feelings and thoughts about illness between, for example, a youth with chronic small bowel disease and one with an absent extremity. The former is likely to distort the condition into primitive fantasies about all internal functions and the personal sense of "goodness" and "badness." The latter generally experiences greatest anxiety because of a direct awareness of physical differences from others.

Prognosis.   The issue of irreversibility has its most profound impact upon the middle and late adolescent and the degree to which the young person may or may not be able to achieve his desired adult role functions. Certainly any condition that interrupts education, threatens vocational goals, or impinges upon prospects for marriage and childbearing becomes critical at this developmental stage.

The older adolescent can generally tolerate immobilization and disfigurement better than his younger peers. But he may experience greater anxiety during illnesses that interfere with the completion of a school year, result in missing important examinations, or force alteration of career hopes.

CASE 10.   An 18-year-old youth severed his right radial nerve when he accidentally put his hand through a pane of glass while playfully roughhousing with his best friend. Although all function returned and he was left with only a residual numbness of his thumb and first two fingers, he became markedly depressed. He had long planned on entering the police force and his disability was now likely to block this goal, as he could no longer accurately shoot a pistol.

CASE 11.   A constitutionally short but sexually mature 17-year-old male had had a great deal of difficulty adjusting to delayed puberty and his relatively short stature in early adolescence and at age 13 had become a heroin addict. Ultimately caught by the police and remanded to a therapeutic community, he finally came to terms with his body image and found a sense of acceptance and self-esteem in becoming a jockey. But the painful knee following a fall off a horse was due not to the suspected torn cartilage but, rather, to an osteogenic sarcoma for which a mid-thigh amputation was indicated. We do not know the ultimate course of this boy, but the crisis he now faces is obvious and the likelihood of a return to his addiction is very high unless vigorous compensating efforts are planned.

Causality.   An issue not often looked at is the patient's factual or fantasied perceptions of his own involvement in the causality of an illness or disability. In many instances it is not uncommon for an injured youth to believe that he is somehow to blame. The guilt engendered by these beliefs can strongly influence behavioral responses. Considering the high incidence of trauma among adolescents and their seeming accident proneness, we suspect that unconscious guilt, self-punishment, and retribution mechanisms are operative in this age group much more frequently than is recognized.

CASE 12.   A 14-year-old boy was admitted for reduction of a fractured humerus. Just prior to being taken to the operating room he suddenly panicked and bolted down the hallway. After he was retrieved and calmed, it became clear that his action was set off by overwhelming guilt and an unconscious fear that the anesthesia was a form of retribution and that he would not come out of it. For not only had he stolen the bicycle he was on when the accident occurred, but he then proceeded to ride it into a little children's playground that he, as an older youth, had been forbidden to enter. Somehow he had managed to get himself and the bicycle entangled in a crash with the jungle gym—and thus fractured his arm.

Not only are there reality-based guilt conflicts as in the case cited above, but accidents and even illnesses may be perceived as punishment for forbidden fantasies in relation to masturbation, sexual daydreams, or thoughts of omnipotence. For instance, an adolescent who develops pneumonia shortly after having entertained aggressive fantasies toward his parents or even openly rebelling against them may feel that there is a cause-and-effect relationship even though there is no realistic basis for such a conclusion. For the most part such perceptions are unconscious and the youth is unaware of these associations; however, they should be suspected in a patient with an excessive degree of anxiety about an illness or injury that is unexplained by other factors.

Another aspect of causality relates to suicide. Whether manifest in an acting-out gesture as a means of securing attention and help or in a genuine attempt to end life, there can be no doubt that a suicidal intent underlies a number of seemingly innocent accidental injuries and deaths. These possibilities should at least be raised in every instance of trauma where the patient seems somehow to have set himself up for the injury. This may be the youth who drives an automobile at breakneck speeds, rides a bicycle the wrong way down a one-way street, climbs on top of a moving elevator, or undertakes some other such hair-raising feat.

On the other hand, we do not wish to minimize normal adolescent experimentation as a frequent cause of trauma. Teen-agers do indeed have a kind of magical view of their invincibility, and undoubtedly the vast majority of injuries are due to such perceptions and the total lack of caution and conservatism characteristic of these years.

A last point that needs to be raised in this section concerns the patient injured in an accident in which one or more friends or family members were also injured or even killed. With the high incidence of multiple-person automotive accidents today, such an event is not uncommon. The added imposition of concern for the injured or mourning for the dead will certainly complicate the adolescent's adaptation to his own situation and will be particularly manifest in depression. If the youth was in fact driving the car or believes he was in some way to blame for harm to family members or friends, matters obviously become even worse.

CASE 13.   A 17-year-old girl and her parents were walking out of a store after having purchased some new bedroom furniture as her birthday gift. A drunk driver lost control of his car, mounted the sidewalk, and slammed into the family. The mother died shortly thereafter and the father and daughter both sustained multiple fractures of pelvis and legs. The father recovered quickly but for a time it was thought that the girl would lose her right leg. Prolonged hospitalization with extensive grafting was required to save it and restore even a limited degree of function. Psychotherapy was a highly essential component of management to help the girl not only contend with her mother's death, her father's injury, and her own severe disability and leg disfigurement, but also to help her cope with deep feelings of guilt. She felt the accident would never have happened had they not been purchasing a gift for her.

Psychosomatic Disease.   Consideration of the nature and impact of disease in adolescence would be incomplete without at least some mention of those physical conditions that are known to have a strong psychogenic component if not firm emotional origins. Such diseases as asthma, ulcerative colitis, duodenal ulcer, and anorexia nervosa occur in adolescence with some frequency. We do not propose to expand further on this aspect of illness but merely wish to raise the issue and point out that the problems related to psychosomatic disease are as operative in adolescence as they are at any other time of life. During the teens, however, management may often be much more difficult, in light of the individuating conflicts of these years.

SUMMARY

In this chapter we have looked at the special meaning of illness for the adolescent in relation to a number of factors: age of onset, duration, course, prognosis, restrictiveness, visibility, causality, and psychosomatic components. We postulate that each of these issues bears a unique set of meanings in relation to developmental tasks and that awareness of this impact will allow for more effective management.

Although we will later expand the point more fully, the need to involve a disabled youth in continued schooling and to provide as much activity geared toward achieving mastery and control as is feasible now becomes evident. The requirements of disfigured teen-aged girls for attentions to make them feel attractive and to reassure them of their continued desirability can be appreciated. Frustrations in contending with the chronically ill adolescent and his sometimes difficult behavior may be more easily accepted. And the crucial need of adolescents to participate in their care and to know what they may expect becomes apparent. At the very heart of the matter is the need of all human beings for relatedness with others and the reassurance that they are loved and loveable and will not be abandoned by those who are important to them.

chapter three

The Implications and Course of Hospitalization

Although obviously a part of the collective impact of other factors of adolescent illness, admission to the hospital and the concomitant implications of this step for the patient are also significant in and of themselves. For the most part, our model for this discussion will be the youth who has had some advance knowledge of his hospitalization, is being admitted for the first time for this condition, and undergoes a diagnostic evaluation, surgical procedure, or medical treatment with good prospects for a favorable outcome. Such a definition will take into account the largest percentage of teen-aged hospital admissions. We will, however, also keep in mind chronically ill adolescents with recurrent or prolonged hospital stays, as well as those who arrive in a state of acute emergency, frequently traumatic in nature.

We do not attempt to define all the possibilities, but rather set forth those factors found to be of particular significance for the majority. Special aspects that apply to the considerably smaller numbers of very seriously ill adolescents or those who are profoundly handicapped are merely touched on here, and are dealt with in depth in chapters devoted to these special concerns.

PRECONCEPTIONS

Everyone has a set of preconceived attitudes and beliefs about hospitals, in both conscious and unconscious terms. Rarely are these thoughts complacent; rather, they tend to be imbued with a sense of both crisis and mystery. In the mind of the prospective patient the hospital is where critical life-and-death matters occur and where the individual comes face to face with major events over which he or she has little control. It is both a place to be born and a place to die; a place of healing and a place of pain; a place of the unknown and alien and a place made heroically familiar by Ben Casey, Dr. Kildare, Marcus Welby, and the other "superdocs" of television.

CASE 14.   A 16-year-old girl was in the hospital for the first time, for evaluation of possible rheumatoid arthritis. Her symptoms were not singularly pronounced and she was reasonably comfortable. After several days she was asked how things were going. She stated that everything was "okay," but that she felt somewhat let down on observing that the hospital was a very routine and ordinary place after all and not a bit like what she had been led to believe from television dramas.

Cultural attitudes also affect this view. The middle-class patient who has received most of his medical treatment in a doctor's private office may think of the hospital in somewhat remote terms, having less personalized feelings about it than the inner-city patient who uses its clinics. In addition, because of the comparative affluence of the middle class, which can afford a wide range of purely elective care, the hospital assumes a benevolent quality for this group and is seen as a source of corrective and cosmetic procedures rather than solely in life-saving terms.

CASE 15.   A 13-year-old girl underwent a cosmetic repair of her nose, which she had felt to be over-large. She had been planning on this for some time and looked forward to the results with both excitement and pleasure. Her mother, an older sister, and a close friend had also had this procedure performed, were most satisfied with its benefits, and had collectively told the patient what to expect. The girl had a most benign and well-tolerated hospital stay.

For those of the inner city, however, the hospital rather than the doctor's private office is likely to have been the primary source of medical attention, and the long waits, depersonalization, and discontinuity so often experienced in clinic and emergency room care frequently instill a good measure of distaste and desire for avoidance. Economic factors for the poor also play a role. Unable to afford the luxuries of elective care or to lose the pay that would result from such an admission and the consequent time away from work, people with low incomes often view the hospital in quite negative and frightening terms as a place where one goes—perhaps even to die—when one can no longer carry on alone. For these people, admission is imbued not only with a sense of fear but also with a sense of helplessness and despair.

Similar associations may be made by rural families when health care is distant at best, both unobtainable and unaffordable except under truly urgent circumstances. Although they may not feel frustrated and alienated, as inner-city residents often do, they may also believe that the hospital is a place to go only when absolutely necessary.

Certainly, personal experiences influence general attitudes. Not only will the individual's own previous admissions be determining (of which we shall have more to say later), but so will those of other family members and friends. Thus the youth whose only direct experiences of hospitals have been with relatives delivering babies will have quite a different set of impressions than the one whose father is in an intensive care unit because of a coronary occlusion.

Similarly, the teen-ager whose best friend had a successful excision of an obvious birthmark or correction of protuberant ears will very likely regard the hospital in much more positive terms than the one whose companion died of a malignancy or following an automobile accident.

Therefore, long before the possibility of admission is ever raised, any prospective patient will have developed certain feelings about it from his own inner fantasies, from television portrayals, from the attitudes of his particular subculture, and from direct experiences in relation to himself, his family, and his friends. Identifying and understanding these preconceptions and taking them into account in managing the hospitalized adolescent is an important first step.

THE HOSPITAL VERSUS ADOLESCENTS

Developmental factors relating to the processes of adolescence itself also contribute to a teen-ager's concepts about the hospital. First, all the social and cultural issues we have just noted are perceived in even more heightened terms. Because of his vivid imagination and rich fantasy life, the youth inevitably responds to the crises and dramas of the external world in an exaggerated way. This will be particularly true in matters that relate as directly to his preoccupation with the body and its functions as do events in the hospital.

From another perspective, being admitted to the ward removes the youth from his or her family, peers, and daily pursuits. It should not be overlooked that the adolescent is, to some extent at least, still dependent upon parents, no matter how vigorous his protests to the contrary. Thus he is not immune from separation anxiety. Further, this is a somewhat more complex matter than for children, involving concerns about being away from the peer group as well as the home. Of course, teen-agers are quite capable of developing an abstract sense of continuity and ongoing relatedness with what they have left behind, and we can expect them to deal with this problem much more successfully than younger patients. However, this may not necessarily be true if the youth has significant doubts about being warmly welcomed by his friends on his return. Such feelings may derive either from past difficulties in interpersonal relationships or from present fears about the alienating effects of the residual consequences of illness or surgery.

Besides separation from family and friends, hospitalization imposes restrictions on mobility, enforces dependence, invades privacy, and threatens autonomous functioning—all critical concerns for an emancipating adolescent. The teen-aged patient's drives for independence are frustrated not only by being confined to the ward and those rules and regulations that curtail his movement, but also by his need to turn to others for even the simplest things that he is used to doing for himself, such as asking for a glass of water, a snack, or an extra pillow. This is further amplified by his having to accept and accede to the ministrations of strangers in such intimate and invasive matters as physical examinations, preoperative preparation, the drawing of blood tests, and the like. If his condition is in fact immobilizing or debilitating to any degree, the application of various autonomy-inhibiting devices—extending from the most sophisticated life support systems to the lowly bedpan, emesis basin, and rectal thermometer—will further compound the confining nature of the hospital itself. The ways in which these measures impede an adolescent's strivings for dignity and independence are clear.

Of course, the amount of anxiety that these issues may generate will be significantly modified both by the seriousness of the medical situation itself and by the individual youth's own developmental stage. In the first instance, concerns about lost autonomy may pale in the face of the threats posed by major illness; in the second, early and late adolescents generally tolerate necessary restriction a good bit more easily than those in their mid-teen years. Under stressful circumstances younger teen-agers return to preadolescent levels of dependency with relative ease, and older youths are much more advanced in securing their independence and therefore are less fearful of losing it. These matters will also be less critical for the adolescent of any age who strongly invokes regression as a major coping device or has primary, unresolved dependency needs arising from preexisting parent-child symbiotic relationships. Such may be frequently seen, for instance, in patients with long-standing chronic illnesses.

Hospitalization and its associated procedures also pose particular problems to adolescent identity development. For the various attendant bodily manipulations are perceived not only as attacks upon drives for independence but also as threats to functional and sexual integrity. Inevitably the enforced exposure of virtually every part of the body, its careful inspection, and its invasion by knife, needle, catheter, speculum, or probe give rise to major fears and fantasies about one's bodily integrity and one's capacity for resuming those activities so essential to adolescent gender and functional role definition.

CASE 16. A 15-year-old boy had been born with penoscrotal hypospadias. Repeated attempts at repair had not been singularly successful, and it was not until he was 14 that a fully normal urinary stream was restored. His most recent admission was for a periurethral abscess and minor scar breakdown, treated by antibiotics and a diverting cystotomy. Although his deep concerns about his sexual integrity had never been directly dealt with or discussed, it was clear that he was profoundly disturbed about this. He was intensely and narcissistically preoccupied with his physical appearance, following a careful muscle building regimen and constantly combing his hair. He had become a neighborhood bully and gang member and boastfully spoke of his multiple dangerous exploits. He also had many girls in what he called his "stable" and was openly proud of his repeated sexual conquests. Particularly difficult to manage on the ward, he was overtly flirtatious with female staff and patients alike, and he complicated his medical course by frequent masturbation that caused further wound breakdown.

The inherent dichotomy between the prime concerns of normal adolescents, on the one hand, and the hospital setting, on the other, sets the stage for major emotional conflicts in this age group. The degree to which a youth effectively deals with this depends not only upon the nature of his medical condition and the inner strength and resources that he can bring to bear, but also in no little measure upon the attitudes and approaches of those who care for him.

THE HOSPITAL COURSE

When the implications of an illness combine with the impact of hospitalization, it is no wonder that most adolescents view such a situation with considerable alarm. But it is also testimony to their resilience and resourcefulness that unless chronically ill, permanently handicapped, or significantly disfigured, the vast majority of teen-agers do very well indeed, adapting to the hospital setting with considerable agility if they are given some measure of understanding and the ward is reasonably responsive to their particular developmental needs. Under these circumstances the adolescent can be a most engaging and enjoyable patient.

On that encouraging note, let us now turn to follow the youth through the course of a "typical" admission and to look more closely at those aspects that are particularly significant for this age group.

The Announcement.   Although ward staff members usually consider hospitalization to begin with the patient's arrival, we have already indicated that in many respects feelings about this started long before, when the child first watched a medical drama on television, overheard relatives talk about their operations, or went to visit a new baby cousin. In more immediate terms, a given hospitalization really begins with the "announcement," that moment in the doctor's office or clinic when the youth and his family are told of the need for admission. The physician's announcement in and of itself implies that the situation is serious, and by the time the youth arrives on the ward an "anxiety set" is already at work and he or she is emotionally geared for action.

The prospect of even minor surgery, albeit seemingly innocuous to the professional, may assume major proportions in the mind of the adolescent. Physicians are not always aware of this, and the particular concerns of this age group are often ignored in preparing them for admission. Teenagers are sometimes not fully informed because of a physician's genuine desire to protect them from being frightened and the mistaken belief that they do not have much more capacity for understanding than do children.

CASE 17.   A 16-year-old girl was admitted for a biopsy of a regional node associated with several thyroid nodules and the possibility of a radical neck dissection if suspicions of cancer were confirmed. The physician had told the patient only of the biopsy but, in order to avoid worrying her, made no preparation for the likelihood of a major procedure. Malignancy was indeed found and successfully removed, but at the cost of major tissue loss and neck disfigurement. Postoperatively, the girl was horrified at what had happened to her and unremittingly angry at the doctor for deceiving her. She was a bright and intelligent girl who quickly figured out that she did in fact have cancer. But, because she had lost confidence in the honesty of those who were caring for her, she refused to accept their reassurances about the likelihood of a favorable outcome that pathology had confirmed. On discharge she became a recluse, appalled by her disfigurement and certain she would shortly die.

All too frequently, many adults (doctors included) have a tendency to regard adolescence as simply a transitional admixture of the qualities of a child and those of an adult, rather than as a quite separate and unique phase in the life cycle with its own purposes and parameters. This general attitude is expressed in the inconsistent position that says to the teen-ager, at one and the same time, "Do as you are told!" and "Act your age!" Thus the youth is not expected to question what is being decided by others on his behalf or to consent to it; he is expected to accept others' decisions, and their consequences, in a mature, poised, and rational manner. Adolescents met with such expectations certainly do come to the ward confused about what is happening to them and why, and what it all means; for their anxieties have usually been neither assuaged nor even acknowledged. In addition, they may be resentful that their questions and thoughts were not elicited or their consent sought in addition to that of their parents. This will be particularly so for those who are highly invested in emancipation struggles.

CASE 18. A 16-year-old youth was admitted for removal of a small lipoma from his back. His doctor had simply announced to him and his mother that it should be taken out and that this would be done under local anesthesia, believing no further discussion was needed. On his arrival, the staff anticipated that this would be a singularly benign admission, as not only was the procedure a minor one but also the boy had the physical development of a football linebacker, and it was expected he would behave in a manner consistent with his appearance. To the contrary, however, he promptly became restless, agitated, and a pest on the ward, repeatedly complaining loudly about such seemingly irrelevant matters as the location and length of his bed and the small size of his television set. It was not until this behavior was discussed with him and his true age and lack of preparation were taken into account that the reasons for his behavior became clear. He expressed what he recognized to be wholly irrational but nonetheless real fears of being conscious during surgery and panic over the prospect of consciously and passively having to let someone cut him open. He was particularly worried over whether he could keep himself from bolting. When matters were explained in more detail and plans were changed to carry out the procedure under general anesthesia, the boy promptly calmed down and thereafter had a smooth and uneventful course.

Although doctors are rarely wholly unresponsive and in general certainly make every attempt to be reassuring, supportive, and optimistic to both parents and youth alike, they may not only unwittingly fail to elicit and respond to the teen-ager's own particular set of concerns, but they also frequently tend to be quite noncommital to all family members about dire possibilities, even if such are high on the list of diagnostic contenders. Thus, for the most part, adolescents with potentially serious conditions arrive on the ward in a state of bewilderment and high suspense, with but only the vaguest of ideas as to what might be wrong and with a host of frightening thoughts.

It is our contention that the youth who enters the hospital fully and honestly informed of why he or she is being admitted, who has been told what to expect, and who has given his or her consent thereto will be far better able to cope effectively than one who has been deprived of such understanding and participation. We do, however, qualify this position for those youths who are to undergo profoundly mutilative procedures, such as amputation of an extremity for osteogenic sarcoma or a colectomy and colostomy for ulcerative colitis. While we firmly believe surgery of this nature should not be carried out without the patient's prior knowledge and consent, just how far in advance of the operation he or she should be told about it is a matter for discretion and judgment. Here the precise timing of talking about these matters will be a much more critical and highly individualized issue than when the anticipated outcome is less functionally disruptive.

Although what actually transpires prior to admission will significantly affect how the youth and his family will deal with the hospitalization itself, it is also important to note that this is a matter the regular ward staff has had no hand in. Thus the adolescent usually comes to the hospital inwardly seething with anxieties and preconceptions unknown to those who will be caring for him. In addition, what had been discussed in advance may not necessarily have been relayed to ward personnel, who will generally have no immediate knowledge of the patient's expectancies about such matters as pain, immobilization, possible mutilation, duration of stay, length of convalescence, extent of recovery, and the like. But it is obvious that if preadmission anxieties have been handled well the youth's ability to adjust will be enhanced, while the converse situation will tend to abet any underlying vulnerability for emotional decompensation. These will be important matters for the ward staff to know.

The Arrival.   While all of the preceding conditions continue to obtain after admission, new experiential components are now added to the total mass of external information and inner feelings that the youth must contend with. In accomplishing this, most adolescents tend to tackle these matters in the same basic ways that they have learned to deal with stress in the past. Indeed, taking a history of such an event often produces information clearly predictive of what behavior may be expected on the ward.

Characteristically, newly arrived teen-agers often seem calm, cool, collected, and rational. They may even appear indifferent. However expressed, the youth's intent is to convey the impression that he is quite in control of the situation, thus masking his inner turmoil. It is wholly consistent with adolescent behavior for the teen-aged patient to affect a façade of being his own master and to give the outward appearance of an adult style of accommodation. This is a direct attempt at preserving a sense of both independence and personal continuity in the face of what is about to happen. Not only does the youth not yet sufficiently know the situation to deal with it more directly, but also what he knows from his preconceptions bodes ill for the preservation of his developmental drives.

It should be noted that these efforts at self-control are generally well received by the staff. Quite understandably, they always find rationality and reason much more desirable attributes in a patient than emotionalism, regression, or belligerence, even though such negative responses may actually be more appropriate behaviors under certain circumstances.

While the preceding is the most common mode of presentation, expectations must be modified for those youths who have evidenced past emotional disturbances and who have thus developed other less felicitous methods of dealing with stress. The boy who tends to respond to difficult life situations by withdrawal, retreat, and regression may arrive on the ward in just such a state. Or the girl who commonly uses manipulative ploys to gain attention she cannot otherwise come by at home may demonstrate such acting-out behavior in the hospital as well and be provocative from the start.

Of course, there are infinite variations on this theme. But one can certainly anticipate that the youth who presents the "cool" façade and is seemingly in control of himself will pose far fewer management problems during his entire course than the one who is invested in avoidance or various acting-out behaviors from the beginning.

One cannot, however, make such predictive statements about the patient who arrives acutely ill or seriously injured. The effects of pain, debility, or significant somatic discomforts substantially alter the picture. Here conservation of emotional energy and a resultant inward retreat are more apt to be the rule. In addition, the possibility of permanent disability or even death is usually appreciated by the youth and he may arrive at the hospital already in a state of grief and mourning. It has been our experience that even when attempts were made to keep such knowledge from a teen-aged patient, he invariably senses the truth, by intuition and from the nonverbal, hidden messages of those about him, for these can never be fully masked. In such instances, it may not be until convalescence is well established and survival assured that even an emotionally healthy patient will be able to mobilize and exhibit his true methods of coping with stress, if indeed he is not so handicapped as to continue to be overwhelmed for an even longer period of time.

Similarly, the chronically ill youth, with a worsening of his condition, may also be expected to have a somewhat different "set" than the norm on arrival. The girl or boy who has been repeatedly hospitalized, particularly if since earliest childhood, may have come to accept hospitalization as an inevitable, necessary, and even reassuring part of his life style. This youth often arrives with a good bit of poise and hospital savvy in knowing just what to expect and how to conduct himself, as well as being familiar and comfortable with members of the ward staff. For others, the admission may represent a discouraging setback or, alternatively, reinforce basic desires to remain dependent. Members of this latter group are much more likely to display anger and hostility or depression and regression, as the case may be.

To summarize, the adolescent's affect on admission is multi-determined in part by his own inherent strengths and vulnerabilities in the face of stress; in part by how he has been prepared for this step in advance; in part by the seriousness of the condition itself and the amount of attendant pain and debility; in part by his immediate perceptions as to his prospects for recovery; and in part by the duration of his illness and what being in the hospital means for his total upward or downward course.

Generally, the ward staff intuits many of these things and attempts to respond supportively. But, without defining what is going on in relatively precise terms, there is always the trap of anticipating that the cool, calm, and collected youth will remain so throughout his stay, or that those who present less acceptable behaviors will inevitably be "troublemakers." Such stereotyping of an adolescent on his arrival always leads to greater difficulties in the long run, for it obscures the normal fluctuations in mood and behavior that will occur during any youth's stay on the ward. If stereotyping is avoided, these shifting moods can to a large extent be anticipated and effectively dealt with.

On the Ward.   Being in the hospital presents each youth with not only a unique crisis but also a very real challenge. At its most deleterious, this will be a time when premorbid immaturities and developmental delays are reinforced. Such may occur when, for whatever reason, the youth has been unsuccessful in beginning his emancipation and unconsciously wishes to avoid entering this state.

CASE 19.   A 17-year-old youth, away in college, was admitted for severe migraine headaches. These seriously interfered with his ability to function and he was forced to return home. While in the hospital he remained in bed much of the time and demanded endless attention. This regressive behavior was quite inconsistent with his medical state.

On further investigation, it was found that the boy was the only surviving child, three other pregnancies having terminated in miscarriage. The parents, fearful of losing another, had always been exceedingly overprotective and had rarely afforded the boy the chance to go out and about on his own. While he did well academically he had few socialization skills. On going away from home for the first time he was ill equipped to meet the new demands in interpersonal relationships and in managing his own affairs. His headaches and immature behavior were effective, although unconscious, ways to force a return to a more dependent state.

Alternatively, hospitalization may simply be a time of transient maturational arrest or temporary regression with a return to normal emotional development on recovery. But, most constructively, the hospital experience can be a time of personal growth and positive gain with the discovery of new strengths in successfully dealing with pain and frustration and in resolving stressful conflicts. This is the goal we would ideally try to help each patient achieve during the course of her or his stay on the ward. It is, indeed, a wholly realistic prospect. To discharge a young person who has coped well with a difficult situation, discovered new inner capabilities and courage, and learned to take pride in these accomplishments is one of the rewards of adolescent medicine.

To define matters more precisely, we can reasonably look at the course of the average adolescent patient as consisting of a progressive series of shifting behaviors and attitudes. We have come to identify these shifts as comprising four phases: "anticipation," "acute reaction," "positive coping," and "resolution." But, before discussing them in detail, we do wish to note that the parameters of these distinctions are blurred. One imperceptibly blends into another and each is highly subject to individual variation. Unless seriously ill for prolonged periods of time or left with serious residual handicaps, the emotionally resilient teen-ager usually progresses through these steps quite rapidly. Most adolescents will have adjusted quite well to their situations within three or four days after admission or following surgery. Nonetheless, we have found the following analysis to be a useful method of "tracking" the patient's course, so that staff need not be thrown off base by unexpected but still normal behavioral shifts. Further, anticipation of what may occur also allows for recognition of the patient's most vulnerable times and permits the prompt institution of preventive or therapeutic measures.

We define the phase of *anticipation* as covering that period during the initial hours of admission when little is happening. At this time, the youth is not singularly stressed by other than routine admission procedures. He occupies himself by collecting as much data from the environment as he can to better assess the situation and calculate just how best to respond. At issue is the preservation, if at all possible, of his sense of personal integrity and autonomy. Behaviorally, this is manifested in the continuation of the controlled pose characteristic of many adolescents when they first arrive on the ward. This is a time of watchful waiting, of sizing things up.

The phase of *acute reaction* begins when somewhat more aggressive medical procedures have been initiated or surgery has been carried out, and extends for a day or two while the imposed onslaught upon the youth's body is experienced, in fact or fantasy, as unexpectedly overwhelming and frightening. The patient who has never before been hospitalized or had an operation is generally unprepared for the reality of confinement, the invasion of bodily privacy, the associated pain and debility of surgery, and the like, no matter how much thought he may have given to this beforehand. These realities are usually totally new, beyond past personal experience. It is inevitable that the youth will be taken off guard to some degree and temporarily set back in working out just how to contend most effectively with the situation in order to regain mastery and control. Of course, medical circumstances often quite realistically require at least a transient abdication from these drives. For being ill, having surgery, requiring intravenous therapy or traction, and so on make anyone more dependent on others. And in particularly serious situations the youth may have an even more difficult time figuring out how to cope to his best advantage.

In this phase some degree of regressive behavior is characteristic, and the adolescent may, to a variable extent, be whining, querulous, irritable, and quite intolerant of pain. He may be the antithesis of his usual self in demanding frequent attentions and ministrations for even the smallest of matters that he could in reality tend to himself. Frustrated by his relative immobility and powerlessness, worried about what is being done to him, in suspense over its outcome, to say nothing of being genuinely uncomfortable, the youth may at times also express considerable hostility, accusing both staff and parents of unconcern and unresponsiveness to his needs. At other moments he may retreat and become sullen. Barricading himself against further onslaughts, he licks his wounds in isolation, unable to mobilize a counterattack upon the insults to his body and those who are inflicting them.

This is, of course, the time when not only are matters most difficult for adolescents to bear but also when young patients may be at their most obnoxious and hard for the staff to tolerate. But a sympathetic acceptance is indicated while responding to the patient's demands in the best way one can, realizing both that they can never be fully met and that this time will soon pass. If such does not occur, there will be time enough to deal with this later on and one should not be impatient. Staff expressions of intolerance and exasperation at such infantile behavior or outright avoidance fails to recognize that the patient has been temporarily disabled, emotionally as well as physically. The consequences of such responses are to aggravate matters further by reinforcing the adolescent's confusion and anger about the assault on his body and feelings of frustration at not being able to control either himself or the situation more effectively.

In most instances, this reactive phase quickly abates when pain and discomfort lessen and the full dimensions of the circumstances become better known and understood. Once the worst of possible test procedures and therapies have been met and endured and the youth is assured that he can in fact survive them without figuratively or literally coming apart at the seams, matters are no longer so overwhelming and decompensating.

At this time the teen-aged patient can be considered to have entered the phase of *positive coping* as he takes up putting his anxieties into manageable proportions through those counterphobic measures and coping devices (chapter 4) that employ mastery and control. By these mechanisms the youth again takes charge of himself and reengages with those about him in positive and age-appropriate terms. However, these efforts may initially be expressed in rather exaggerated terms, as the adolescent often becomes melodramatically effusive. Seeking to be the center of attention, he often looks for the continued approbation of others in confirmation of just how well he has survived these events. These actions basically serve to reassure the youth that he has not been irreparably mutilated or functionally impaired beyond what he can contend with and that his capacity for peer group acceptance, ability to attract opposites, and assertions of independence can be as they were before. At times the demands of this somewhat manic behavior, even if good-natured, can also be difficult for the staff to contend with. In addition, this hyperactivity can act to the youth's own detriment if it interferes substantially with required bed rest. But here, too, understanding the intent of such actions and responding to them in a flexible and reassuring way will be considerably more effective than the rigid and unperceptive imposition of repressive measures.

As convalescence progresses and recovery begins, the youth more and more comes to sense that he has successfully passed his crisis and that he is not substantially changed. He perceives that whatever defect he may now have can be satisfactorily integrated into his body image without any serious deficit to his former concepts of self and feelings of self-esteem. It is this awareness that constitutes the phase of *resolution*. At this time the collective impact of the illness itself and the event of hospitalization are integrated into the patient's personality, and he resumes his normal progress. Ideally, his development will have been augmented and enriched by having met and conquered a major life stress well.

MODIFIERS

Throughout this discussion we have primarily considered the course of the emotionally intact youth who has come to the hospital for a relatively short stay and returns to good function. We have, however, alluded to various exceptions to our "model." At this point we shall review and expand these modified circumstances, consolidating them under one focus.

Chronic Illness.   As we have noted, the patient who has had a long-standing illness with remissions, exacerbations, and repeated hospitalizations arrives on the ward with a quite different emotional set than our "typical" youth. In many respects he is an old hand at the business of being ill; he knows his way around. Unless past experiences have been singularly painful or unusually unpleasant, he will have relatively few apprehensions about the hospital experience itself and his primary concern will be weighted far more on the side of what admission means for the course of his illness.

Indeed, for some, being on the ward may be more comforting and reassuring than not. A youth with a debilitating or disfiguring condition, who finds it both taxing and depressing to try to keep up with his normal peers, may feel much more relaxed and reassured in a setting where everyone else his age is also ill and where he can compete on comparable terms. Further, if he has felt poorly much of the time and has had to strain to keep up with his schooling and other daily tasks, the hospital may be a haven and refuge where he need not struggle so hard. Finally, if the chronically ill youth has been dependent on parents and others to care for him or if his family have been overprotective, warranted or not, his emancipation may well have been delayed. In such circumstances the hospital frequently serves as an extension and reinforcement of what has become a comfortable *modus vivendi* in being cared for and remaining dependent.

On the other hand, if the adolescent's development has not been handicapped by continuous illness and if his course has been one of only infrequent exacerbations, having to be admitted may represent quite another matter. For he must again face the disconcerting fact that he is not normal. Here the hospital raises the specter of continued poor health with all the concomitant limitations on one's prospect for a full and complete life that this implies. Such a youth has a realistic basis for being depressed, angry, hostile, or withdrawn or having any one of a number of other negative attitudes and feelings.

CASE 20.   A 17-year-old-boy had undergone uneventful surgery for aortic stenosis at age 10. However, he experienced this as an extremely painful and frightening time and was intensely relieved when he was told that he was well. Thereafter allowed full activity, he participated happily in all athletics. But at age 17 he was found to have developed aortic insufficiency and cardiac enlargement with early signs of decompensation. His activity was immediately curtailed and a valve replacement urgently recommended. The boy's response was one of bewilderment, and panic, resulting in an inability either to eat or to sleep without sedation. He was angry at those he felt had duped him into believing he was well. He was afraid he would die without an operation, but he was unwilling to subject himself to another horrendous surgical experience. Faced with this dilemma, he did not know which way to turn.

In such instances the phase of "acute reaction" is frequently prolonged or even fixated, and the management of the chronically ill adolescent represents a major challenge to the ward staff. The passive, dependent patient needs to be helped to enter into the individuating processes of adolescence to the degree that his condition permits. The resentful, angry, or rebellious teen-ager needs to be provided with all of the constructive, compensating activity that can be brought to bear. For both, the basic goals are to provide a milieu in which they are nonjudgmentally accepted and cared for, yet in which unacceptable behavior is clearly defined; to promote self-care and self-responsibility to the greatest extent possible; to encourage peer group interaction with other patients on the ward; to promote visiting by friends and family; to support continuation of schooling and appropriate vocational plans; and to teach new skills consistent with the patients' handicaps through which they can develop autonomy, mastery and control, and self-esteem.

It must be recognized, however, that some adolescents will have illnesses so debilitating or handicapping that they are profoundly invalided. One cannot always hope to construct a relatively normal existence for these youngsters or avert some degree of emotional invalidism. Just how limited they truly are must be carefully and realistically assessed, and as meaningful and rich a life as is possible under the circumstances must be developed. It is sometimes a very hard task for the staff to accept the reality of such profound limitations. Not only is it painful to see a young person denied any reasonable prospect for fulfillment of his childhood promise, but this also brings professionals square up against their own fallibility. But not to deal positively with things as they are and either to continue to offer unrealistic hope or to avoid coming to grips with matters at all, just letting time slide by, may result in the patient and his family never coming to any constructive terms with the situation at all. In consequence, the youth may passively wait for an improvement that may never occur, or for an early death that does not arrive.

CASE 21. A 14-year-old girl was diagnosed as having lupus erythematosis with renal and cardiac involvement. Her prognosis was poor, and a kind of fatalism set in among those who cared for her. Although treatment maintained her in a relatively ambulatory state, her frequent school absences and easy fatiguability caused her to drop out and to remain at home all day, doing nothing but watching television. After about two years she surprisingly remitted and was deemed quite capable of returning to school. This was easier said than done. The abdication of her physician from a positive coping attitude and the expectations of her family that she would die within the first year had resulted in a universal abandonment of any attempts at all to make the most of whatever quality of life was available to her. These attitudes could not be changed and although still in remission at age 19 the patient was an emotional recluse, unable to leave home, engage in social activity, or perform any job function. The physician in this instance was one of the authors (A.D.H.) early in her career.

Serious Trauma.   Every adolescent ward has its share of teen-agers who are admitted following a serious accident, often with major neurological and/or orthopedic sequelae. For automotive- and sports-related accidents and trauma resulting from violence are collectively the leading causes of both morbidity and mortality in this age group.

At the time of admission, the patient is often unconscious or, if conscious, in an obtunded state of awareness because of emotional and physical shock. Even if he is aware of his surroundings, the youth is far more preoccupied with the terrible insult to his body and its associated pain than with whether he is in the hospital or not. If he considers this matter at all, he is likely to see the hospital in highly protective terms and to experience little if any sense of frustration or anxiety about being there.

Certainly, at this critical stage—when the saving of life and limb and the alleviation of pain are preeminent—it is inappropriate to be preoccupied by the psychological impact of the moment. Concern for a patient's emotional integrity at this point in time is somewhat irrelevant to the reality of the situation, to say the least. Later, when life is assured, the injury stabilized, and the true extent of permanent injury more apparent, the implications and meaning of the situation become a primary concern. This shift of focus occurs not only in the minds of rehabilitative staff but also in the mind of the victim. Even though the patient may not be especially verbal on this point, it should not be overlooked. Patients are often afraid to ask for confirmation of what they sense is true, and it is important not to be fooled by their seeming lack of interest.

Where prospects for good recovery are real, the patient quickly picks up the optimism of those about him and then frequently follows the typical course. However, he or she may continue to have anxieties about the accident itself and to be phobic about the circumstances of it for some time. But when a favorable outcome does not appear to be in the offing, the youth senses this not only from his own inner perception but also from the distress of his parents and the hospital staff, no matter how vigorously cheerfull their pretense may be. It is not unusual for such a patient to progress through the phases of hospitalization very slowly, with months or even years between the reactive and resolution stages, if indeed the latter is ever fully achieved.

To cope meaningfully with a serious unremediable disability is extremely difficult for the adolescent patient. It is also difficult for the staff, who must contend with their own feelings about seeing a teen-ager's future imperiled and about being unable to offer significant help. The tendency of both is simply to avoid discussing reality in constructive terms. This offers neither party any real solutions and only perpetuates a frustrating and unhappy stalemate.

CASE 22. A young resident was both bewildered and upset about how best to manage three teen-aged boys with recent spinal cord injuries who were all in the same room together. Two were paraplegic and one quadriplegic. Medically stabilized and their survival ensured, the boys were just beginning to sense the full extent of their injuries. Their tentative questioning about whether they would ever walk again created considerable staff anxiety and consternation about how to respond, and by and large these queries had been parried and put aside. The resident spoke of his overwhelming wish not to have to go into the room each day. He could not help his own countertransference and feeling that for the quadriplegic youth, in particular, death might have been a better alternative. For several hours after each visit the resident felt pervaded by depression and frustration that genuinely interfered with his effective functioning on the ward. But, when these matters were brought out into the open and reality-based prospects for rehabilitation reviewed, a much less emotionally disabling situation ensued.

Obviously, these are most difficult situations to deal with in any terms and there are no easy or set answers; this question will be dealt with further in chapters 10 and 11. The issue is raised here, however, to complete the spectrum of the impact of hospitalization.

The Emotionally Disturbed Adolescent. It is an important matter to differentiate between the teen-ager who is normally labile with rapidly changing and shifting moods and the one who is disturbed in the true meaning of the word. The former, if not faced with permanent alterations of body function, generally has a favorable emotional outlook, although the ward staff may have to scramble a bit in helping the patient achieve this goal; whereas the latter will frequently pose vexing problems for himself and others throughout his course.

The emotionally troubled youth inevitably brings his difficulties with him onto the hospital ward, just as he has brought them to other crises in the past. These may or may not relate to previous illnesses. But, regardless of the genesis, a teen-ager who in some way feels short-changed by life and is consequently angry and hostile will inevitably demonstrate these feelings on the ward. So, too, the youth who is chronically depressed or the one who has learned that recognition and attention only follows manipulative and provocative behavior will often recapitulate these patterns at this time.

CASE 23.   A 14-year-old girl was remanded to the hospital by the courts for treatment of pelvic inflammatory disease. On admission and throughout her stay she was depressed, sullen, and clearly hostile. Indeed, it was difficult to secure her cooperation for even the simplest of diagnostic and therapeutic procedures. Further history revealed that she had been bounced from one foster home to another, always rejected sooner or later for temper outbursts and lack of lovability. Most recently she had been placed in a juvenile shelter from which she had run away. She was found living with a young man in his mid-twenties who rather regularly beat her up when she failed to take care of his creature comforts. She was a profoundly disturbed youngster whose behavior patterns derived from a deep-seated and well-founded mistrust of others. Throughout her stay she continued to be suspicious, isolated, and easily angered. Efforts to involve her in psychiatric treatment failed. On discharge, she again ran away and was heard from no more.

Emotional problems—except those engendered by the current medical condition itself—generally antedate hospitalization, and hard evidence of such difficulties can usually be found in the history. Indeed, in many instances, identification of such matters will be critical to understanding otherwise confusing responses to hospitalization itself.

CASE 24.   A 13-year-old boy was rendered unconscious in a bicycle accident. After a period of time he regained consciousness and seemed well. However, his thinking processes continued to be somewhat disoriented, his verbal output impoverished, and his behavior immature. It was thought he might have sustained more brain damage than was originally believed. On reexamination of the past history, however, it was determined that he had long been limited in his mental ability and had attended school only through the fourth grade. Further, according to his parents, his present behavior was not significantly altered from what it had been before his accident.

Regrettably, information on psychosocial functioning is not always obtained routinely. Unexpected behavioral problems all too often start things off on a bad footing with a resultant unnecessary crisis on the ward. Thus, a critical component of management is the anticipation of maladaptive behavior, which then allows for the development of a meaningful therapeutic response, rather than simply succumbing to a clash of opposing wills in confrontation over what the staff may view as perverse and stubborn behavior.

CASE 25.   A 17-year-old boy, diagnosed as having cavitary tuberculosis, was admitted to an isolation unit and placed on appropriate chemotherapy. History revealed that the youth had long had difficulties in tolerating frustration with major problems in impulse control. He had dropped out of school in the tenth grade after being frequently truant for many years and recently had left a Job Corps placement after only a brief stay, as he felt this to be too regimented. It was immediately anticipated that major difficulties could arise about treatment continuity, maintenance of isolation, and possible elopement. But it was also known that he was deeply concerned about his own health and about possibly exposing his family and friends. Indeed, he really did want to cooperate with treatment. When these factors were all taken into account, the adolescent medicine fellow provided close and continuing supervision and support, coupled with empathy for the boy's feelings of frustration. A recreational worker developed as much of a diversionary program of mastery and control as was possible under the circumstances. The teacher worked with him toward a high school equivalency diploma that he wanted. And the staff was not particularly distressed when he did in fact elope, as they calmly had anticipated this and predicted he would soon return—which in fact he did. On discharge, the youth remained under the care of the adolescent medicine fellow who had a good relationship with him. This was deemed particularly important as the instability of his past behavior suggested that he might also have major difficulties in sticking to a prolonged but necessary regimen of daily pill taking.

It is our position, then, that the routine search for possible past emotional difficulties and the conduct of a psychosocial inventory (see chapter 8) is just as much a part of the total adolescent patient evaluation as is the identification of strictly biological problems. Not only is this essential to developing a program that allows for optimum compliance with medical management, but it also provides the basis for helping the youth to develop more constructive patterns of behavior. It should always be kept in mind that the adolescent ward can be a psychotherapeutic milieu as well as a place for biological care. When staff offer continuing acceptance, support, and encouragement of the healthier aspects of a patient's behavior, while yet setting limits on his more maladaptative patterns, much redirection can be initiated. At the core is helping the disturbed adolescent to find a sense of self-esteem through positive coping mechanisms and to discover that he need no longer engage in acting-out or isolating activities. In our experience this goal has been realized with sufficient frequency as to make this a practicable aim and not just wishful thinking.

FAMILIES AND FRIENDS

Up to this point we have looked at matters largely from the perspective of the adolescent. But the youth does not function in a vacuum. The experience of hospitalization inevitably has its impact on other family members and close friends as well. Although we look at these persons in concluding this chapter, their interests and concerns, both in terms of their own needs and their effect on the patient himself, are matters to be considered from the beginning.

Parents.   There is no question that the hospitalization of an adolescent is as much a crisis for his parents as it is for himself. All the preconceived notions about the hospital with its associated fantasies and fears are theirs as well. And, while parents are not so stressed on issues of independence and identity, and do not need to face directly the bearing of pain and discomforting procedures, they do have special difficulties of their own.

First, parents' deep natural concern for their offspring's well-being is often further colored by strong feelings of guilt that they are somehow to blame for the situation through neglect. This may be particularly acute in adolescence, for parents always take calculated risks when they grant, or have been forced to concede, increasingly greater freedoms and independence to their teen-ager; and they know full well that he faces considerably greater potential for harm than before. Also, if intrafamily communication is less than open, as may well be the case during the teen years, the youth may not reveal symptoms of illness to his or her parents until it is quite advanced; parents may thus blame themselves for not knowing their child was ill and for not taking action sooner. Certainly the self-recrimination that mothers and fathers experience when their child is ill is no less when the child is an adolescent than when he is an infant or a toddler. Indeed, it may well be aggravated by the fact that the youth is in greater risk and in poorer communication than he was in younger years.

Second, parents may also have ambivalent feelings about their teen-ager's hospitalization. On the one hand, they certainly do not wish to see him sick or hurt, and they certainly look forward to his return to good health and normal development. On the other hand, they may also enjoy the reestablishment of that more direct nurturing role that they have been in the process of giving up in the face of their adolescent's emancipation. This can be a particular problem for mothers who have found their primary meaning and purpose in being a child bearer and rearer. Having to relinquish this role is indeed threatening. The opportunity to set this task aside and to resume a comfortable and familiar identity through taking care of a sick adolescent—made childishly dependent again by his illness—may be welcome. The possibilities for preserving this state indefinitely through overprotectiveness are indeed tempting.

From the opposite vantage, parents who have developed new roles as their adolescent has grown up and away may find it difficult to again resume a nurturing relationship. Simply being at the hospital a good bit of the time may be sufficient to present a problem. The mother may, for example, now have a job, and both parents may be involved in new activities. Such parents also may experience ambivalent feelings, but here the conflicting factor is a measure of resentment at having a situation thrust upon them that represents a regression in and imposition upon their own personal growth.

Another problem faced by some parents is when they are privy to diagnostic and prognostic information that, for one reason or another, is to be withheld from the youth. It can certainly be difficult, if not impossible, for mothers and fathers to attempt to keep up a cheery, encouraging, and optimistic façade in front of their teen-ager when they know he is to undergo some mutilative procedure, has a potentially fatal disease, or will never regain normal function. (Parenthetically, we reiterate that, although we do recognize that parents should often know of these things before their offspring, we do believe that sooner or later the patient should also be told in terms he can deal with and understand. These matters can never really be hidden. Further, the opportunity for an open dialogue among the parents, the adolescent, and the ward staff about the true state of affairs allows for an honest sharing of each other's feelings, greater mutual support, and an ultimate resolution that will always have more meaning, dignity, and strength than can ever be created by continued false pretense.)

Last, while the patient is usually allowed a goodly measure of emotional regression, parents are generally expected to be stalwart pillars of strength and not to add to the burdens of the staff by being demanding or in the way. Indeed, an old familiar adage can be rewritten to read "A parent should be seen and not heard" as far as the pediatric ward is concerned. Mothers and fathers of hospitalized children are not infrequently regarded as necessary encumbrances to the process of making the juvenile well. This difficulty can be even further compounded when teen-agers are concerned. This derives from the natural empathy staff members usually experience for those they care for, often functioning as advocates and defenders of the patient in opposition to his adversaries. As adolescents quite often put their parents in this category during the height of emancipation struggles, the staff may tend to side with the youth and unwittingly project like feelings of impatience and intolerance toward his family. The parents, of course, will be both bewildered and distressed by these quite subtly and unconsciously transmitted negative attitudes on the part of the staff. And, when such feelings are exacerbated by lack of communication with a formerly close and affectionate child, the feeling of being excluded, an alien outsider on the adolescent ward, may also be another singular problem that parents must face.

Siblings.   Frequently, brothers and sisters of the hospitalized patient are simply ignored during the whole transaction. For it is quite true that they play little visible part in the total scene and may not even come to visit. But one needs to keep in mind that siblings are also subject to substantial anxieties about what is happening. Aside from their genuine concern for the well-being of the patient is the disruption and alteration of their family life: one of its members is missing and their parents' attention is directed elsewhere. This will pose little problem during the average hospital stay or where siblings are not very young. However, when extended hospitalization is required, or the other children are still quite little, some attention must be given to the effect this is having on them and their own possible feelings of loss or neglect.

Peers.   As we have noted, peer group membership is critical to adolescent development. In some ways, friendships with members of the same and opposite sex are of equal importance to a teen-ager as his relationships with his family. At times they may be even more important. Thus, close friends, and the dating partner in particular, have a major vested interest and deep concern in the patient's welfare in the hospital. Yet, being outside the family constellation, they are often excluded from the hospital experience. Such exclusion not only ignores their own needs but also denies the patient the special support they may give. Thus we stress here the importance of involving close friends, speaking with them, keeping them informed and recognizing that in them the patient may have firm and resourceful allies in the business of getting well. For it will be the teen-aged peer who can best reassure a handicapped or disfigured youth that he or she will not be cast out and ostracized and that he or she is still a welcome and wanted friend.

CASE 26.   An 18-year-old male was hospitalized for severe recurrent osteomyelitis of his right knee. Indeed, amputation was being considered. Understandably, the youth and his family were very depressed and discouraged about his failure to get better. One or the other of his parents was with him for most of his waking hours in solicitous attention. Finally, expressing considerable exasperation at their over-protectiveness and "babying," the youth asked the staff to keep his parents from coming so often and to arrange for more frequent visits from his girlfriend. She had felt awkward in the presence of the patient's mother and father and had come but rarely. When his wishes were carried out, he became much less depressed and was far better able to cope with his condition.

CONCLUSION

In this chapter we have looked at a number of factors that contribute to the meaning of hospitalization for an adolescent, his family, and his friends. We have also tracked the teen-aged patient's course as he moves from admission to discharge, examining some of those issues that may modify this "typical" pattern. These matters add one more building block to understanding adolescent patients and the particular concerns from which our management approach is derived. It is, however, always important to keep in mind that in defining these issues we have of necessity resorted to categorization and classification. But every patient is unique, possessing his own particular set of responses that differentiate him from every other patient. Certainly, no two teen-agers exhibit precisely the same patterns of behavior, just as all teen-agers do not grow at precisely the same rate. At the same time there are broadly definable developmental parameters for normal youths in general, as well as specific needs that are common to ill adolescents as a class. We have attempted to examine these matters and to establish some basic precepts that will still allow for individual variation in their application.

chapter four

Coping with Stress

Up to this point we have been largely concerned with the impact of illness and hospitalization upon adolescent development. But of equal importance and certainly of more direct interest to the ward staff will be the kinds of behavioral responses these stresses may evoke. Whether the youngster is helpful and cooperative, gives everybody a hard time at each turn, or retreats and isolates himself are obviously critical matters. How constructive behavior may be reinforced and maladaptive behavior deterred is, indeed, what this book is all about.

Let us begin to examine this issue by considering those intrapsychic methods by which the patient may defend himself against stress. Admittedly, this chapter offers a somewhat simplistic view, and we wish to note at the outset that coping behavior is considerably more complex than we indicate here and that substantial controversy still exists in the precise classification of a number of these responses. Nonetheless, we have found this pragmatic view to be a practical and useful scheme for those professionals and paraprofessionals who deal with the hospitalized adolescent on a day-to-day basis. An understanding of coping mechanisms both allows anticipation of the average adolescent's behavior during hospitalization and provides a basis for analyzing the situation when things do not go well. From such an understanding may come a comfortable and logical management approach.

In theory, when an intervening crisis, or stress, disrupts psychological balance the resultant disequilibrium inevitably produces anxiety. This in turn serves as an internal alerting device, stimulating the unconscious to attempt to regain intrapsychic comfort. The various ways in which this is carried out, successfully or unsuccessfully, are often called coping mechanisms. The choice of which mechanisms will be invoked and the timing of their operation are unconsciously determined by the interaction between the inner meaning and impact of the stress itself and the precrisis psychological patterns and resources of the person involved. This sequence of events is normally operative in the process of adolescence itself. Successfully coping with the developmentally generated conflicts, stresses, and anxieties of these years is part and parcel of maturation.

These same principles also apply in the crisis posed by illness and hospitalization. How this particular stress is dealt with in terms of which coping mechanisms are called upon and how they are applied determines the patient's behavioral course and, further, establishes whether the youth remains psychologically intact, fixates at a particular developmental level, regresses, or, optimally, gains maturity and finds new inner strengths. The dual goals of management should be to enhance the patient's use of the more constructive mechanisms and to attempt to turn aside the more maladaptive. It should be kept in mind, however, that certain of the less felicitous responses are often transiently normal at certain points in an illness and therefore should be tolerated and accepted even if they are temporarily counterproductive.

Insightful Acceptance.   Of course, the most constructive and ideal response to illness is by insightful acceptance. In such a situation the individual comes to view the condition itself as quite separate from his estimate of inner self-worth and without any sense of resultant personal devaluation. However, this is a highly unlikely prospect for any person at all points in the course of a serious medical condition. It is even more unlikely in an adolescent who is at the peak of narcissistic bodily concerns, sees his acceptance by others largely in terms of his physical appearance, and has not as yet developed a secure sense of self-esteem. Therefore, insightful acceptance of physical disability is not a readily available alternative for this age group without a lengthy adjustment period.

Denial.   As applied to illness, *denial* may be defined as a complete and quite straightforward intrapsychic disclaimer that a disease, its effects, its implications, or other discomforting aspects of the individual's experience exist at all. This device is probably the most common one employed early in the course of a serious illness, and it is frequently at work in the long and sometimes harmful delays that often occur between the appearance of significant symptomatology and the patient's seeking medical care. Denial may also be a paramount causative factor when a patient fails to keep appointments, forgets to take medication regularly, or otherwise does not comply with recommended treatment.

Obviously, in these circumstances denial is hardly constructive. Satisfactory adherence to therapeutic plans can often be accomplished only when both the adolescent and his family give up this mechanism and come to accept the situation as it is. Thus a vital component of medical care rests in recognizing when this device is operative and in helping the patient to move away from it, at least to the point where it does not seriously interfere with essential treatment.

CASE 27.   A 14-year-old boy was admitted with a large neck mass that was later diagnosed as Hodgkin's disease. This highly visible and enlarging lesion had been present for several months but had been ignored by both the patient and his family. This occurred in spite of his viewing several television dramas wherein the very symptoms were recapitulated in a person of the boy's own age in exquisite detail and in spite of the parents' full intellectual awareness of the implications of this mass for their son.

In a number of situations, however, a certain degree of denial may be appropriate and even helpful, particularly when it is applied in an isolated manner to rather dire but still distant prognostic potentials or other serious implications of disease that neither medicine nor the patient can do anything about at the time. A diabetic youth, for example, who refuses to accept the very real likelihood of a significantly shortened life span but who is still able to follow the prescribed medical regimen may find this device very useful in handling otherwise overwhelming thoughts. Because it allows hope—and thus the continuation of normal maturation and enjoyment of life—constructive denial can be a key component of medical care.

Intellectualization.   Well known to health professionals, who themselves use intellectualization as a major defense against anxiety, this psychologic device separates rational thoughts about disease from the affective aspects of its impact. The latter remain repressed while the former are dealt with quite consciously. Thus mastery and control of the situation, and hence reduction of anxiety, are achieved by focusing solely on the academic and practical side of the matter. In most instances this mechanism serves all concerned quite well; indeed, it is a mainstay of patient-staff interactions. Perhaps at times it may even be used to excess, prohibiting the patient from ventilating his very real fears. However, intellectualization generally allows for excellent medical management and effective patient functioning.

Adolescents who intellectualize rarely "make waves" on the ward. Further, because this academic approach is highly esteemed by the medical profession, these patients are often more favored by the staff than those who have frequent emotional outbursts or little apparent rational interest in their condition. The resultant harmonious relationship provides the youth with yet additional support.

The adolescent who is culturally geared toward scholastic achievement is particularly apt to use intellectualization, often asking innumerable questions and voraciously reading anything and everything about his condition he can get his hands on. This may present problems, as the books and materials that a youth most often has access to are those in school and public libraries. Such publications are notoriously inadequate. Not only do they often distort the real state of affairs, because of literary license or ignorance of the lay writer, but even if factually sound they are usually quite out of date, presenting the patient with a welter of confusing misinformation. Thus it is well for the physician to advise of such problems and pitfalls and to provide the adolescent directly with honest and up-to-date information in a hopeful and positive manner.

Of course, intellectualization has its problems. As we noted in chapter 2, the ill and anxious adolescent easily distorts factual material. The inner emotional meaning of a given illness, even though repressed, cannot always be totally ignored. Inevitably the youth becomes unconsciously caught up in unrealistic fantasies and fears and distorted body-image concepts. This may lead to heightened anxiety and the collapse of intellectual defenses.

It should also be recognized that what appears to be intellectualization may in fact not be such at all but, rather, an indirect and highly acceptable way of asking questions about one's continued attractiveness and acceptability to others or of seeking reassuring attentions in countering fears of abandonment and even death. The youth about to undergo heart surgery, for example, who expresses keen interest in his cardiovascular function and physiology and in precisely what the procedure will involve, may be invoking true intellectualization. But it is also a strong possibility that he is really seeking reassurance about his survival, while at the same time making sure of the continued firm interest and concern of those staff members upon whom he must utterly depend to survive.

Intellectualization, then, may at times be a most effective defense and one to be promoted. It is particularly useful in those situations where full recovery is anticipated or where the illness is stabilized without substantial impairment of function or appearance. However, it may also be a fragile, deceptive device, and its usefulness is probably more circumscribed in those conditions where there is a significant permanent loss of mobility or major disfigurement. Under such circumstances intellectualization must also be accompanied by genuine ventilation during a period of open grief and mourning or order to work through the loss and come to a more enduring resolution.

Rationalization. Closely related to intellectualization, this mechanism is manifested in passive acquiescence to a situation that is seen as inevitable. The patient adopts the fatalistic view that it is beyond his ability to do anything about the illness anyway and what happens is completely out of his hands. In this manner he extricates himself from experiencing anxiety by accepting the condition in a detached and unchallenging way.

CASE 28. In a tractor accident a 17-year-old farm boy had avulsed his entire right brachial plexus, resulting in a flaccid paralysis of his right arm. With no prospect for return of function, an amputation was ultimately carried out so that a prosthesis could be substituted for what had become a useless and awkward extremity. The youth expressed an extraordinarily calm and fatalistic acceptance of this highly mutilative procedure, stating, "I know it will never get better and what has to be just has to be. These things just happen on the farm sometimes anyway, and I'm lucky to be still alive."

As in this instance, rationalization can be a useful device when it is based in reality: when a disability is in fact unremediable and permanent or when prolonged periods of hospitalization are required, as in the treatment of bacterial endocarditis, severe scoliosis, and the like. These situations must indeed be rationalized and accepted. But it is obviously unconstructive when a patient remains fatalistic beyond the dictates of reality, abandoning efforts to get well and succumbing to invalidism, when to the contrary his or her prospects for improvement or recovery are good.

Rationalization is relatively infrequent in adolescence. Any mechanism that relies on a passive, fatalistic acceptance is quite antithetical to the teen-ager's strong, instinctive developmental drives for autonomy and self-determination. Rather, it will be much more commonly employed by parents in an attempt to cope with their own anxieties over their offspring's illness.

Regression. This mechanism is, as the term implies, a moving backward to an earlier developmental level. In adolescence it is a time of abdication from continuing the developmental tasks of these years and a return to an earlier state of childhood dependency. In this way the patient no longer need bear the burden of anxiety and fear himself, but instead hands it over to parents or their surrogates to manage. At times, especially when regression is abrupt and unexpected, the staff may be confused, as when a youth, previously invested in emancipating struggles, suddenly begins to clamor for attention, does not want to be left alone, and prefers his parents' presence to that of his peers.

Quite normal in the early phases of illness or injury, regression is universally encountered in response to pain at any time. In the initial days of hospitalization, when the condition is acute, or when surgery has just been carried out, regression is not only characteristic but also appropriate. Bedridden, uncomfortable, and feeling poorly, the patient does need to be taken care of and is indeed more dependent than before. To attempt to be autonomous while encumbered by intravenous tubing, oxygen tents, and other life support systems, as well as by the debility of the condition itself, is hardly realistic. Further, there may even be a temporary enjoyment of regression in succumbing to the seduction of normal parental oversolicitousness and heightened attentions during their child's illness.

However, as convalescence progresses and the patient begins to feel better, the emotionally healthy youth abandons this mode and resumes his former developmental drives. Problems with excessive or persistent regression occur mainly when the condition realistically requires prolonged or extreme dependency, when it directly interrupts a vulnerable stage of adolescence, or when preexisting psychopathology has already impeded the adolescent's normal quest for autonomy. In the first two instances regression can usually be worked through with time. But particularly where an unhealthy degree of premorbid parent-child symbiosis and parental overprotectiveness have substantially antedated the current hospitalization, regression may be much more pervasive and difficult to deal with.

Another group of adolescents who also may have considerable difficulty in giving up regression are those who, instead of being overprotected, have been emotionally deprived for much of their lives and seek an infantile type of nurturance in all their interpersonal relationships. When such a youth becomes ill, his or her profound inner dependency needs may become ascendant. This is most evident in the youngster who wishes to stay in the hospital even after he is quite well. To a more normal degree, this mechanism is also operative in the young person who keeps returning to the ward to visit long after medical treatment has been terminated.

Reaction Formation and Compensation. Some degree of compensation is almost always used by emotionally healthy people in response to illness, particularly during convalescence. It is probably the most effective adaptative device short of the idealistic prospect of integration, sublimation, and insightful acceptance. In an effort to regain self-esteem and resume a measure of mastery and control, the patient substitutes positive and usually constructive counterphobic behavior for behavior that is no longer physically possible.

Compensation is a highly useful and desirable method of dealing with chronic disease or permanent disability that compels a youth to change his or her usual activities. A newly handicapped adolescent who previously sought his or her identity through sports, dance, or other such vigorous endeavors may come to find acceptance, achievement, and individuation through the alternatives of scholastic performance or artistic creativity in learning to play a musical instrument, paint, or become proficient in handcrafts. Compensation is clearly operative when a disfigured girl designs and makes her own attractive clothing to hide her deformity. Also, various alternative physical activities may be substituted for those that can no longer be performed; a boy who can no longer participate in rough contact sports might substitute track, tennis, or golf.

In short, this mechanism works through constructive, substitutive methods of maintaining a sense of purpose and place. In the adolescent it continues to provide opportunities for the furtherance of mastery and control and for role definition. The stimulation and provision of compensatory activities is a critical component of managing hospitalized youth.

Projection.   Through projection, one's own feelings are unconsciously held to derive from others. This device is commonly used in response to a patient's mounting anxiety due to believing that he is somehow to blame for his own situation. The resultant sense of despair, personal disgust, or self-anger is averted by holding someone else to be at fault instead. The patient need no longer acknowledge his own responsibility and experience guilt once he has managed to convince himself that fault rests with another. Adolescence provides particularly fertile ground in which opportunities for projection may spring up. Not only is there a high incidence of self-incurred injuries secondary to teen-aged experimentation but also any illness in these years bears a firm potential for being unconsciously seen as punishment for the many forbidden fantasies normal to youth. Projection is particularly likely to occur when a youth first becomes truly aware of the full implications of a serious condition and finds his feelings of anger and rage at his fate more than he can bear.

The patient may vilify parents and hospital staff members in accusatory outbursts about their unresponsiveness to his needs, their lack of concern, or their outright failure to provide "necessary" or timely care. A common example is the youth in pain who quite regularly berates the nursing staff for purported insensitivity and unwarranted delays in responding to his or her requests for analgesia or other comforting ministrations. (Of course, regression may be operative here as well.) Obviously such outbursts make it not only difficult for persons who are their target to continue to help, but they also quite effectively block more constructive methods of coping. If such behavior remains persistent and unyielding to staff efforts at promoting more positive and productive mechanisms, the intervention of a psychiatrist, psychologist, or social worker is indicated. However, the transient appearance of projection may be just as inevitable early in the course of a serious illness or accident as are denial and regression, and it should be understood, tolerated, and worked through as such.

Projection may occasionally have legal consequences as well. It is not uncommon for a disabled patient to impute, without real cause, his disability to the negligence of the hospital staff. Thus, projection is often at the heart of many unfounded liability suits and malpractice actions.

Displacement and Isolation.   Another common coping device is the unconscious transfer of intense anxiety and concern about oneself onto some other more emotionally distant and manageable matter. Displacement is frequently employed during illness and hospitalization—for there are many times during the course of a major disease when the patient has little or no control over what is happening to him and thus simply must tolerate the resultant anxiety. Curtailed drives for self-control and self-determination may at times leave displacement as the only positive, adaptive option available to a youth attempting to stay on top of the situation.

It is no easy matter for a patient to cope with mounting fears of the unknown while waiting for test results, waiting for doctors to decide what the problem is and what to do about it, waiting for surgery to be carried out, or waiting for the disease itself to take its course. Under such circumstances, it is constructive to displace the intense concerns about oneself, which one can do nothing about anyway, onto some other matter over which one has at least some degree of mastery and control, even if it seems irrelevant and trivial. Thus adolescents about to undergo major surgery may seem calm and coolly indifferent toward their impending operations and yet be highly preoccupied about missed schooling, hospital food, problems of a roommate, whether their parents will take adequate care of their pets or possessions while they are away, and other such unrelated matters.

CASE 29. A 17-year-old girl was hospitalized for a rash and a fever of unknown etiology. She appeared seriously ill. Numerous tests were carried out over many weeks in a futile, frustrating effort to differentiate between the leading diagnostic contenders of collagen disease, malignancy, and sepsis. After a six-week course of unremitting spiking fevers, she got well spontaneously. During her entire hospitalization she never expressed any interest or concern in her condition and blandly and passively accepted the numerous and often painful test procedures without question or protest. In contrast she became frantic over the possibility that she might fail her upcoming college board examinations and spent all the energy she could muster in studying for them, despite the fact that she was an excellent student and the teacher had reassured her that she would surely pass with flying colors under any circumstances. A number of months later she was finally able to verbalize that she had really thought she was going to die and had been deeply terrified by the obvious and quite genuine concern of her doctors about the gravity and perplexity of her diagnosis.

Displacement, then, is by and large a useful coping mechanism. It allows for the diffusion of even major levels of anxiety without interfering with either medical care or meaningful interpersonal relationships. Indeed, recreational therapy firmly encourages patients to employ displacement as the first and simplest line of defense. Every hospital has, at the very least, its volunteer cart of assorted bedside activities. Friends and family intuitively encourage displacement when they bring the patient books, magazines, or games. The youth who can be involved in reading a good novel, putting together a craft kit or jigsaw puzzle, listening to records, playing cards, and so on can focus his energies in diverting activities and perhaps forget his problems for a while.

Displacement may be "person-directed" as well as "object-directed," as when worry and anxiety about oneself is converted into an altruistic concern about the worries and anxieties of others. Such displacement, however, is usual only among youth who have already progressed from the narcissistic stage of sexual role definition to a more mature level where they are developmentally capable of mutually shared affection. It is primarily the late adolescent, then, who, suffering a serious or even terminal disease, is able to concern himself about the well-being of his family and to attempt to protect them from distress over his situation. We have seen such youths even extend this concern to include the feelings of the hospital staff in expressing appreciation for their efforts.

Other examples of person-directed displacement are not unusual. A youth who sustains a major illness or serious injury may express gratification that it happened to him or her and not to the girlfriend or boyfriend who is deemed more vulnerable and less able to cope. A hospitalized teen-ager may help to take care of other more acutely ill patients on the ward. In this way the young person not only manages to displace her or his distressing thoughts and feelings but also to enhance a sense of mastery, control, emotional strength, and self-esteem.

Albeit useful, displacement is nonetheless a quite superficial device, reflecting more a holding action than anything else. Thus, while it is effective in handling relatively short-term stress, particularly when awaiting major medical events, it has limited value in matters of longer duration. In instances of chronic illness or permanent disability, the consequent anxiety inevitably rises to the surface sooner or later and demands a more permanent and effective adaptation. Optimally, this will be compensation, if not genuine insight. With time and the support of the ward staff, initial displacement may indeed be converted into such modes.

Acting Out.   In acting out, the patient deals with threatening matters through inappropriate and often negative physical activity. Technically, this is a form of displacement, but is set apart here because it is essentially maladaptive rather than constructive. At its core is either an irrational desire to escape from the situation or an unconscious, manipulative attempt to secure reassurance of one's self-worth not forth-coming by other means. Consider the little child who provokes inattentive parents to spank him because even such painful attention and contact is better than no contact at all. Coping mechanisms of this nature are often most difficult to contend with and frequently culminate in a management crisis on the ward. Indeed, under some circumstances it can become a critical matter to provide even the most basic medical care.

Acting out may be manifested in a variety of provocative behaviors such as sexual aggressiveness, verbal abuse, elopement, outbursts of anger, physical attacks, refusal to cooperate with treatment, actual sabotage of care, and so on. Often, if the past history of the youth is known, similar responses to other earlier crises or past difficulties in impulse control will be readily evident, as the following case so dramatically illustrates.

CASE 30.   A 15-year-old girl had swallowed half a dozen straight pins, one of which had been aspirated and had required a thoracotomy for removal. Her postoperative course was uneventful and the remaining pins passed on through the gut without difficulty. Subsequently, it was learned that she was beset by troubles at home, that she had swallowed the pins deliberately, after an argument with her boyfriend, and that she had acted similarly on a number of previous occasions, although never with such dire medical sequelae. The first episode had been an accidental swallowing while sewing and holding pins in her mouth as a matter of convenience. But the resultant drama, concern, ambulance ride, and hospitalization had been unexpectedly rewarding emotionally, particularly as she had felt fine throughout. Subsequently, she had resorted to this device whenever she felt overwhelmed or rejected. The present episode was the fifth within two years.

Regardless of whether acting-out behavior represents a characteristic pattern of behavior, as in the preceding case, or whether it is a unique response to a singularly overwhelming situation, the hospitalized adolescent who copes in this manner is indeed seriously disabled. To manage such a patient effectively and help the youth avail himself of his more positive and adaptive inner resources presents a true challenge to the hospital staff (see chapter 9).

Unfortunately, instead of calmly implementing a rational plan to deter acting out, hospital staff members tend to react impulsively, first with a flurry of rational appeals and then—when these fail, as they inevitably do—with a firm no-nonsense disciplinary approach or even scare tactics vividly and uncompromisingly describing the dire consequences that are sure to follow if the patient does not behave himself immediately. Such techniques are doomed from the beginning, as they take no account of the underlying reason for the behavior and the fact that it unconsciously arises from irrational fear, true impulse disorders, or well-entrenched and long-standing maladaptive patterns of gaining attention and reassurance.

The staff's failure to control the situation by these methods results only in mounting frustration. Doctors, nurses, and others caught up in the matter may also inaccurately feel that the patient is aiming his anger, hostility, and provocations directly at them in an unwarranted and ungrateful rejection of their efforts to help. How human and understandable it is for a professional to respond to these circumstances by various counteraggressive and even punitive measures. Obviously, when the past history suggests a potential for acting out, careful advance planning is essential. Developing some basic guidelines to be followed when a situation of this sort suddenly crops up is far more constructive than merely "playing it by ear" and risking an intolerable situation of confrontation or mutual abandonment.

CASE 31.   A 13-year-old boy, reputedly "difficult" to manage at school, was admitted for treatment of osteomyelitis of the distal phalange of his right thumb. The initial injury was incurred by an errant hammer blow during his shop class. The infection was quite advanced and required surgical débridement and the institution of a six-week course of intravenous antibiotics. After the first few days the youth found it increasingly difficult to tolerate the relative immobilization and isolation from his peers that the therapy and hospitalization imposed. His anxiety was further heightened by overhearing frequent medical discussions held outside his door as to whether part of his thumb would or would not have to be amputated. Finally he could bear it no longer, smashed the intravenous bottle on the floor, pulled out his needle, and took off down the hall. Retrieved by security guards, his struggling, pummeling, and colorful language were temporarily quelled by chlorpromazine. This cycle of events repeated itself a number of times over the next few days and was countered at first by rational appeals and later by increasingly angry statements from his doctors to the effect that he would be sure to lose his thumb if he did not comply. At the end he was placed in restraints and sedated around the clock. Fortunately, the situation was retrieved through the intervention of a liaison psychiatrist in assisting the boy to ventilate his deep fears about bodily mutilation and the ward staff to develop a more understanding and constructive approach.

Withdrawal.   This reaction is an emotional isolation and walling off of one's inner self in an effort to retreat from and shut out the external threat or stress. Of course, withdrawal is rarely selective. Positive feelings and relationships are likely to be shut out along with painful and depressing matters, rather like throwing out the baby with the bathwater. Thus, emotional isolation cannot often be considered an effective device except in those highly acute, physically overwhelming, or painful situations where the patient's total energies must be directed solely toward biological survival. Under other circumstances, however, withdrawal represents an abdication from attempting to cope at all.

In its typical manifestations, a patient first expresses a diffuse and all-encompassing rage at the circumstances that engulf him; then, when this is expended, lapses into grief and depression; and finally descends into various degrees of withdrawal. In its most intense form, it may be quite difficult to reach such a youth by either verbal or nonverbal means; he may be sullen and distant even to the point of turning away or shutting his eyes and pretending to sleep when a staff member or visitor enters the room. It is hard for such a person to avail himself readily of the comforting support of others (although this is precisely what needs to be offered), to say nothing of participating actively and constructively in his own care. Generally he will be passively compliant even though he may well refuse active cooperation.

CASE 32. A 19-year-old youth had been experiencing progressive neurological and endocrinological symptoms for several years. Two earlier evaluations for possible brain tumor had been completely negative, but a third clearly delineated a mass subsequently found to be a rare, slow-growing teratoma in the region of the pituitary. This was successfully removed. Although he had been quite apathetic before the operation, it was expected that matters would substantially improve once the intracranial pressure was relieved and his moderate panhypopituitarism was corrected by exogenous hormone administration. Over the succeeding two months, however, even though ambulatory and mentally intact, he continued to remain profoundly depressed and withdrawn. Although he allowed his body to be manipulated in any way necessary without the slightest protest, in no way could he be induced to swallow either food or medication. Instead he would simply hold whatever was given him in his mouth for hours on end. Ultimately, it became necessary to create a gastrostomy.

Obviously, withdrawal is not only unconstructive in dealing with stress but may also be dangerous and pathologic if it persists. Nonetheless, it is transiently encountered in many patients. Certainly some degree of withdrawal is most appropriate in response to the depression that inevitably occurs on realizing the seriousness of a disease or its grave prognostic implications. Withdrawal is also a normal response to pain, debility, or discomfort in protecting the individual from the very real assault of illness or injury upon his body. An adolescent, or indeed any patient, may also respond with this mechanism if expected visitors fail to come or upon missing important events in his life, losing a term at school or college, or discovering that he must indeed alter his career choice. He may also become depressed and withdrawn over the failure of surgery to accomplish as much as was hoped for, or upon realizing that an injury will leave permanent and disfiguring scars.

Under such reality-based circumstances, transient withdrawal, frequently accompanied by regression, is an understandable and normal initial defense. It is certainly a more tolerable reaction for all concerned than the other coping device often employed in this situation: projection. As a temporary measure withdrawal should be accepted and understood for what it is, while one continues to encourage the patient to reengage in human contacts and in his usual activities. As withdrawal is generally inconsistent with the drives of the emotionally healthy adolescent, these modes will usually be given up as soon as the youth feels better, avails himself of more constructive outer-directed coping methods, and is able to resume at least some of his normal pursuits. Major degrees of persistent withdrawal, however, are inconsistent with good adaptation and may well warrant definitive psychiatric intervention.

Panic. Of all responses to stress, panic is inevitably the most disabling, both to the patient trying to maintain his emotional equilibrium and to the staff attempting to provide medical care. Not only is the patient rendered helpless, but often the staff also feel overwhelmed and tend to respond in the same counterproductive efforts that they may employ in attempting to deal with acting out.

In its most profound manifestations, panic is a response to an overwhelming stress in a totally decompensated flight-fright-fight reaction. We all know of the classic circumstances of mass panic and hysteria when large crowds are imminently threatened by fire or other such disasters. In the individual, problems of this nature may normally be encountered during altered states of consciousness as during the induction or recovery from anesthesia. With intact cerebral function, however, panic represents a complete breakdown in adaptation. Fortunately, this is uncommon among adolescents. But it may be encountered in patients with preexisting low-stress thresholds or other emotional problems related to impulse control (see case 31) as well as in those faced with an overwhelming reality situation.

CASE 33.   An emotionally healthy 16-year-old girl had sustained a serious crush injury to her leg in an automotive accident. In the emergency room, while being readied for surgery, she overheard the doctors talk to her parents about the very real possibility of having to amputate. Up until this time she had been quietly withdrawn and acquiescent to all that was being done to her. But now she suddenly began screaming incoherently and struggled violently until sedation took effect. Happily, her limb was saved and the girl did very well postoperatively. But she continued to remember vividly and painfully the sense of overwhelming panic and the uncontrollable urge to escape that engulfed her on suddenly learning that she might lose her leg.

As illustrated by this case, no amount of explanation or rationalization can deter the terrifying feelings of panic. Instead, simple statements of reassurance coupled with immediate sedation is the initial treatment of choice. Psychotherapeutic agents such as chlorpromazine or diazepam will help blunt the overwhelming anxiety and place it in somewhat more manageable proportions. Panic is, in our estimate, the only maladaptive behavior discussed in this chapter that nearly invariably should be responded to with prompt medication. Tranquilization may well be indicated under other circumstances but should be induced only after careful consideration of all the factors involved and as but one part of an overall therapeutic plan.

CONCLUSION

Although we have individually described the various unconscious methods by which patients cope with the emotional stress of illness, the picture is rarely so clear-cut. Not only may several mechanisms be operative at the same time in a given individual but they may also occur sequentially, arising at different points in the hospital course.

The selection of any particular set of devices is a matter of some complexity. It is influenced not only by the nature of the illness itself and the real or fantasied meaning of this for the patient and his future, but also by his usual premorbid methods of coping with life stresses, his inner strengths and resources, and the nature of the support and guidance he receives from parents, peers, and hospital staff. In conjunction with this, we must also consider the developmental phases of adolescence itself and the various specific vulnerabilities of the early, middle, and late teen years. We should also recognize that even within the confines of these given periods maturation is a halting and somewhat erratic process. Thus a youthful patient may be reasonable, helpful, cheerful, calm, and cooperative—invoking compensation, intellectualization, and constructive denial—at one moment but may become depressed, disruptive, demanding, and manipulative—exhibiting projection, depression, regression, and acting out—at another, simply because he is an adolescent.

In our experience, however, it has not been difficult to pick out the most significant operative coping mechanisms and basic strengths for any given patient and to arrange his milieu and gear his management toward supporting the healthier of these modes and minimizing the less constructive. Indeed, we will suggest in subsequent chapters that for the vast majority of patients such will follow almost automatically from applying a basic set of age-appropriate management principles in a ward setting that is "tuned in" to needs of adolescents in general.

chapter five

Ward Staff Interactions among Themselves, Patients, and Parents

Staff interactions—both one to the other and in conjunction with the patient, his family, and his friends—are vital determinants of effective management. A well-defined and coordinated ward team will face far fewer difficulties in caring for the adolescent patient than the one with blurred and isolated functions and fragmented communications. This is particularly important for teenagers, who become easily confused by mixed signals, frequently distort information received from a variety of independent sources, and engage in highly exaggerated fantasies when they do not know just what is going on. Under these circumstances, behavioral problems are all too apt to occur. But we post fair warning that the development of such a unified approach first requires a critical analysis of customary management modes. This inevitably will raise some harsh and perhaps painful truths.

STAFF TO STAFF

Doctors. We cannot deny the existence of pecking orders and hierarchies in the overall ward system and in its component disciplines. These rank downward from various grades of experts to novices to students. Senior attending physicians and private doctors are at the top, functioning as the directors and controllers of patient care. The remainder of the hospital staff are, in many respects, cast in supportive and subordinate roles, carrying out the doctor's orders and making the patient as comfortable as possible in the process.

Further, the primary physician, unless he or she is an intern or resident, is generally not a member of the permanent ward staff and is not consistently present to direct patient care. Rather, she or he visits the floor, sees the patient, writes any desired orders, and leaves. Information exchange with other professionals is frequently scanty, often accomplished only through brief chart notes. There may be few opportunities for sharing such matters as long-range plans; what has been conveyed to patient, family, or others; prognostic implications; or discharge plans. Of course, the time that this takes poses real problems for the busy practitioner. And it is also true that the practitioner may have problems in securing the attention of other staff members when they make their rounds. Nurses, interns, and residents, occupied elsewhere with other matters, sometimes view the private doctor's arrival as disruptive of their own routines.

The roles of house staff officers tend to be more ambiguous than those of novices in other disciplines. For the private patient, this is an apprentice relationship wherein interns and residents simply carry out orders, monitor the patient, alert the private doctor when problems arise, and act on their own initiative only in emergency situations. There may be major problems, however, when a bright new medical school graduate wishes to be more aggressively involved in directing care. This is particularly likely if he disagrees with the private physician's management. While it is well within his function to question such matters in an intellectual search for knowledge away from the bedside, he nonetheless is expected to continue to follow the attending doctor's orders, or find indirect ways of implementing his views.

This is in marked contrast to interns' and residents' relationships with ward patients; here they usually serve as the primary doctors themselves, under the aegis of a senior attending physician. While the latter may function in either an advisory or directive role, depending on the philosophy of the service involved, in all training programs these junior staff members assume considerably more responsibility for ward patients than they do for private ones. Of course, communications are far easier under these circumstances as, for a time at least, these persons are assigned to the ward as their sole duty and are readily available to others for much of the day.

On the other hand, the rotational nature of house staff training programs poses its own set of difficulties in providing continuity of care. This will be confusing both for the hospitalized patient, who may see a number of residents and interns come and go during his course of treatment, and for the discharged patient, whose care may be handed over to a clinic physician whom he or she has never met. All too obvious is the confusion that may be experienced by a ward patient trying to figure out who his or her primary physician is. A further problem posed by the rotation of house staff is the matter of physician commitment. An intern or resident who sees the end of his term on the ward looming over the horizon tends to relax his grip on difficult situations, waiting for the time when he can hand them on to his successor. Conversely, a new arrival, recently rotated and inbued with zeal, may reinstitute heroic investigations and efforts that duplicate or confuse what has already been done.

Medical students on the ward but further confuse patients in trying to figure out just who's who. Much of the "doctor time" for both ward and private patients is spent with inexperienced students, who often have much more personalized and less disciplined relationships with them than other staff members do. Discomfited by a certain sense of charlatanism in posing as graduate physicians, most students also display a somewhat hesitant professionalism. Yet ward patients, in particular, tend to regard these young, interested, and highly attentive future physicians as the ones they can rely on most and may turn primarily to them for support and answers to their questions. The adolescent patient further complicates matters by being singularly apt to relate to and identify with the medical student who is closer to his own age, is considerably less authoritarian than others, and usually offers the fewest difficulties to youthful emancipation drives and efforts to retain control. Reciprocally, medical students are often highly empathetic to adolescent patients and sensitive to their needs because of this very closeness in years. Yet in so many ways this group is the least well equipped to manage teen-agers and the most likely to overidentify and become pawns to the patient's manipulations.

The need for a medical or surgical specialist-consultant on a case further complicates the hierarchy. This generally poses little change in the traditional *modus operandi* for private patients; the specialist and the attending physician are usually in close communication, functioning as a unit. But where nonprivate patients are concerned, care often tends to be taken over by specialty senior residents or fellows, with major lapses of communication as a consequence. This is particularly apt to be true when the specialist and the resident or intern assigned to the ward are from different departments (e.g., surgery and pediatrics). Interdepartmental information exchange and coordination are far more of a problem for medical specialties than for other disciplines that are not so compartmentalized.

CASE 34.   A 14-year-old boy with Marfan's syndrome had been hospitalized for surgical treatment of recurrent retinal detachment. Frightened and confused, he had been deeply concerned about what was happening and his prognosis. The adolescent ward resident had been unable to contact the boy's ophthalmologist, who had, in fact, not spoken to the boy or his family at all. In addition, major questions relative to his discharge remained unanswered, such as school return, permissible exercise, participation in sports, and other such matters. One morning the boy was gone. His discharge was unexpectedly ordered by the ophthalmologist the night before, and his then visiting mother had taken him home. A telephone call revealed that the family had still not received any answers to their questions other than the fact that the surgery was "successful." The boy did not even have a return clinic appointment.

A word also needs to be said about the traditional role of the psychiatrist on the medical ward. The tendency has been to call in this professional only when emotional matters have gotten clearly out of hand, such as psychotic behavior, threats of suicide, or flagrant acting out. In these instances the psychiatrist's function is specific: to evaluate the situation and take over management through tranquilization, treatment, or transfer. Usually, however, scant thought is given to the psychiatrist's general function in enhancing staff capabilities for dealing with patient problems or for helping them to understand and more effectively cope with their own anxieties. Certainly little emphasis is placed on the whole concept of preventive mental health for both patients and staff.

Nursing.   Nurses are traditionally expected to play a much more supportive and less directive role, carrying out the physician's orders and tending to the day-to-day needs of the patient. Of course, they do have a certain degree of autonomy. Often functioning *in loco parentis,* nurses have considerable control over the patient, and they exert authority over most other professionals on the ward, exclusive of physicians. However, although nurses are central in the total functioning of the ward, they have not usually been allocated any major decision-making functions. Perhaps in no small measure reflecting male chauvinism, the relation of nurses to physician has long been viewed in the same light as wife to successful husband—"the power behind the man."

Thus, nurses have long been in professional quandary: they often know considerably more than others about their patients as people, because of a unique closeness to them, yet they are given little opportunity to contribute to patient planning or to make direct management recommendations to physicians. Of course, nurses have also long managed to find ways out of their predicament, circumventing the problem by offering suggestions obliquely and indirectly. Nevertheless, doctor-nurse relationships do need to be reexamined and realigned—horizontally rather than vertically—so that the best of the skills and knowledge of each can be openly shared and applied without the barriers of traditional hierarchies.

There is a no less rigid autocracy within nursing itself than within medicine. In many respects the members of hospital nursing staffs have even less independence and are more locked into fixed procedural pathways within their own discipline than are doctors within theirs. While the latter tend to function relatively autonomously, each from the other, nurses at one level are much more subject to the authority of those on the level just above. Thus the nursing supervisor is considerably closer and more directive to ward head nurses than a department chief is to his attending doctors. Further, many nursing functions are largely pre-determined by a highly detailed and quite inflexible set of rules, regulations, and memoranda that have been compiled over the years and collated into the procedure manual.

Such a system does have its strengths, genuinely allowing for optimal communication between various members of the nursing staff and their various shifts. Further, it leaves little to chance and minimizes error. However, particularly insofar as adolescents are concerned, this system also has its problems.

There is no more fatal pitfall in caring for this age group than attempting to apply a fixed set of routines and procedures. Confrontations and power struggles are the inevitable consequences. Inflexibility is often the precipitating cause of a "behavioral" crisis on the ward. Indeed, the causes of such problems can far more often be traced directly to hospital rigidities than to any inherent "obstinacy" on the part of the teen-ager himself.

Flexibility toward adolescents within the nursing sphere is perhaps far more critical than for any other group of professionals involved. Because of the intimacy and constancy of their contact, nurses are the primary responders to an ill adolescent's reality-based dependency needs, and they may come to be viewed as symbols of lost autonomy and control. To assist a young person to see matters realistically, to avoid distorted fantasies, and to cope effectively, rather than to rebel or retreat, requires considerable nursing imagination and initiative.

Recreation and Education.   Recreational, occupational therapy, and educational staff are rarely considered as integral to the functions of the ward. In many hospitals there may be no secondary school teacher at all, and recreation workers may simply be kindly volunteers who help while away the time or bring diversional reading and craft materials to the ward. Even if such personnel are more professional, their disciplines are often still seen as functioning somewhere beyond the pale of the patient's "real" medical and nursing needs. They are considered as time fillers rather than as constructive and critical adjuncts to the development of positive coping mechanisms and a return to optimal function. In some instances the work of these professionals may even be impatiently viewed as merely interfering with the business of the day, such as when the patient a doctor has come to see is off in the schoolroom or participating in a recreational event. Certainly teachers and recreational or occupational therapists are rarely included in or informed about overall therapeutic planning. Their functions are thought to be at best peripheral and at most secondary to the process of getting patients well, if they are even thought of at all.

Social Workers.   In the overall picture, social workers have also had a secondary and mechanical role on the ward. Tradition has held them to be mainly advisers to the family at times of financial crisis and bureaucrats who carry out referrals to other agencies and institutions. In conventional terms, the social worker helps to get indigent persons on welfare, arranges for postdischarge placement when needed, manages school and vocational difficulties relative to the patient's illness, obtains funding for special appliance, and the like.

Social work intervention is often deemed necessary only for the economically disadvantaged, and these professionals may not even be assigned to a floor unless a significant number of patients there are poor. The contribution that social workers can make to the daily functions of the ward and its total mental health through ongoing emotional support of the patient and his family, regardless of their economic status, and through contributing to and sharing in comprehensive long-range planning is often quite overlooked.

Others.   The hospitalized patient also encounters a wide variety of technical-support and housekeeping personnel. While these people may play a critical role in the hospital experience of many patients, they are generally quite removed from participating in coordinated planning. Communication with these other staff members is largely through written orders, requisition slips, telephone calls, and written reports. Yet the singular importance of the nutritionist to a youngster with diabetes, the radiotherapist to one with a malignancy, or the physiotherapist to a paraplegic is obvious; and the omission of these specialists in team planning and coordination can be a weak link in comprehensive care. Nor can one ignore the effect of a housekeeping aide who grouchily chides a youth about the mess at his bedside or complains that his slowness in eating regularly delays her picking up his tray. Contrast her with the bright, friendly aide who enters the patient's room with a smile and is not upset if she is put off her schedule a bit.

Clergy.   This group of professionals is frequently not only overlooked, but frankly often ignored. For the most part, health care providers relate to patients in a highly intellellectual way, with little regard for spiritual needs. Even though assigned full time, in many hospitals members of the clergy usually function independently of other personnel, making their own rounds or being called in only at the request of the patient himself. Rarely are they included in deliberations about patients, even those with strong religious ties, and the resulting lack of communication can sometimes have distressing consequences.

CASE 35.   A 14-year-old boy was admitted for the surgical correction of a minimally disabling spinal deformity. He was clearly a religious youth, with a crucifix and rosary attached to his bedstead. Unbeknown to the ward staff, the hospital priest visited the youth the evening before surgery. As there apparently was some question as to whether the youth had ever been baptized, the priest performed this sacrament. The next morning, on arrival in the surgical suite and while being transferred to the operating table, the boy suddenly panicked, leaped from the stretcher, and cowered in a corner, terrified. The procedure was canceled and the patient was returned to the ward. Further investigation revealed that the youth had fully appreciated the unspoken message inherent in his being baptized; so that should he die he would not be deprived of the opportunity to go to heaven. Indeed, of all messages received, this was the most powerful and over the night his unbridled fantasies distorted the precautionary nature of this act into the firm conviction that he would not survive surgery and that the priest was the only person being fully honest with him. Had the clergy been included in total patient planning, this event might have been avoided.

STAFF TO PATIENT

In this context we define *staff* as collectively consisting of all those professionals mentioned in the preceding section, and characterized by providing some sort of direct service to the patient. And, although there will be variations in the precise nature of the staff-patient relationship from one discipline to another, there are certain themes common to all. First, to be truly satisfying, all jobs must have their own emotional rewards as well as economic gains. For health care professionals such gratification derives in large measure from the pleasure of being wanted and needed. To this end we often have definite expectations as to the ideal patient. As pointed out by Vistosky and his co-workers, we tend to differentially reinforce and favor friendliness, appreciation of staff efforts, patience, understanding of the many demands on our time, a sense of humor, an attitude of optimism, and belief in self-improvement through effort.

We have observed that pediatric staff tend to look for these virtues in parents, while accepting and welcoming the child's dependency, perceiving themselves as subsitiute parents and perhaps even better than the real ones. Of course, these attitudes inevitably present problems in caring for the ill adolescent who has neither the emotional maturity to live up to those expectations set for adults nor, in his striving for emancipation, the capacity to be dependent as a child.

In addition, many professionals tend to feel that the ideal patient should also be an acquiescent and passive recipient of care, even to the point of being overdependent at times. Patient passivity is not only consistent with the staff's own view of their dominant, caring role, but it also represents the behavioral posture that is least likely to obstruct the performance of procedures or to interfere with the maintenance of "discipline" on the ward. Individuality and self-assertiveness on the part of the patient are often seen as disrupting this balance. Yet the repression of these latter attributes is quite antithetical to the developmental drives of young people, and expectations of acquiescent passivity may frequently be unrealistic and will often form the nidus for confrontational power struggles.

A further point here is that the ward staff frequently tends to view adolescents as younger than their real developmental age insofar as their capacity for self-determination and self-responsibility is concerned. Hence, compliance is often sought through a parental and controlling approach at one moment and, when this fails, as it inevitably will, through cajoling and bargaining at the next. On the other hand, this view of teen-agers as children does not usually extend to expectancies about how they will act, and adolescents are concomitantly supposed to be rational and reasonable and to behave like adults. This attitude, which says to a teen-ager, "Do as you are told, but be grownup about it," is obvious in its inconsistencies and can only be confusing, if not frankly alienating, to the youth who is expected to abide by it.

Secrecy is another common characteristic of staff-patient relationships. There is generally a great deal of reluctance toward telling the patient much of anything about the precise nature of procedures, test results, medications, and the like. Further, hospital personnel tend to be quite reticent about fully informing the recipient of their ministrations on what is going to happen in advance or explaining why, and rarely tell him as much as he would like to know. This attitude goes hand in hand with the staff's own view of themselves as benevolently paternalistic and of the patient as a passive recipient of care. And, while matters may be conveyed in a bit more detail to parents or other close adult family members, here too much will be left unsaid. In consequence, the patient and his family are frequently deprived of a substantial amount of information that they have both the need and the right to know. We see this as perhaps an honest but misguided attempt to protect the patient from being unnecessarily upset, or simply as an accommodation to a busy and hectic schedule that does not afford the time for such explanations. But, more unconsciously, ignorance is also an excellent method of keeping the patient dependent and compliant. For he cannot question, or challenge, or protest what he does not know.

A last point, already alluded to, is that institutions and many of the staff members who serve them are unfailingly rigid. Hospitals are notorious for subscribing to a firm and fixed set of rules and regulations wherein the specific needs of patients become subsumed to the general need of the institution for control, uniformity, and predictability, as well as for the protection of its own legal skin. While we do not deny that these matters are important to the smooth and efficient running of a large hospital, we deplore the fact that in consequence the patient is all too often dehumanized, or at the least forced into an alien conformity, as the following examples demonstrate.

CASE 36.   Rectal temperatures of all patients in a particular hospital were taken four times a day. No one seemed to know quite why this was so frequent for even those who were afebrile. It had "always been that way" and was a requirement set forth in the procedure manual. But the rectal thermometer was used, not because it was deemed to be more reliable, but because several years before a senile patient had bitten the oral type in two, cutting his tongue, and his family had sued.

CASE 37.   The adolescents' recreation room was located one floor above and directly over the ward itself. Although it was but a single, short flight of stairs or a quick and nearby elevator ride away, no patient, no matter how ambulatory, was allowed to go there without being escorted by a staff member. Parents or friends would not do. The teen-agers complained that not only were they inconvenienced, as escorts were not always available when they wanted them, but that they were also humiliated by this demeaning precaution. The hospital administration was unyielding because of the possible legal liability should any injury come about in transit.

CASE 38.   Several adolescent rooms had recently been opened at one end of a pediatric ward. Up to this time the evening visiting hours had been over at 7:00 P.M. and lights had been turned out at 8:00 P.M., an appropriate time schedule for younger children. Efforts to have these hours extended for the adolescents in conformity with those set for older patients elsewhere in the hospital failed. Administrators said that such differential privileges would be "unfair" to the littler ones and that the change would be unacceptably disrupting to the usual evening staff routines.

CASE 39.   A 17-year-old high school senior was admitted for evaluation of asymptomatic weight loss. It became increasingly clear that her workup would require her to stay longer than expected, causing her to miss a college scholarship examination. The girl requested a pass to take it. Although there were no medical contradictions to this, there were no administrative provisions for a patient's leaving the hospital for part of a day and the nature of the legal liability involved was unclear. Her request refused, the patient and her family were forced to sign out against advice.

It cannot be denied that traditional staff-patient roles and relationships often tend to work against the teen-ager, failing to take developmental requirements into consideration. We suggest that most hospitals and their staffs have a set of expectancies that are not only irrelevant to the needs of this age group but that may actually be repressive and inhibiting to an adolescent's best efforts to get well.

STAFF TO PARENTS

We have already looked at some of the relationships between staff and parents in exploring the implications of hospitalization in chapter 3. Our remarks also obtain here. In particular, we wish to reiterate that if staff unilaterally ally themselves with the patient, either as a better parent substitute or as an overidentifying youth advocate, there will be inevitable competition with the true parents and a resultant struggle for control over who is really in charge and who cares the most. Mothers and fathers are often seen as impediments to ward functions, rather than as collaborators in the care of their child. This view is clearly evident in those pediatric systems where the hours for parental visitation are strictly limited.

Although the nonrevelatory attitude of staff toward patients may be somewhat less toward families, there is still the tendency to ignore them, if possible, or to turn their questions and concerns aside with only the briefest response. Much of this predicament stems from the fact that no one is really comfortable in imposing painful, frightening, or disfiguring procedures on another, even though necessary. Especially where children and adolescents are concerned. When parents are present or know too much, the possibility of their expressing undisguised and uncontrolled anxiety not only threatens to upset further an already distressed child but no less to undo the professional's own defenses. Staff may also fear the accompanying possibilities of outright parental emotional decompensation, resistance to and sabotage of treatment, or even physical intervention in procedures. Obviously, concern for such eventualities piles further stress upon the staff. This is most effectively precluded simply by barring parents from the scene as often and as long as possible. Families are not always regarded as helpful reservoirs of strength and support that can be constructively tapped, even though this may be the case more often than not.

From the parents' point of view, it is difficult to stand back and see relative strangers minister to their child and perform functions that they hold to be their own. In addition, they must allow and even support the deliberate hurting or even mutilation of their offspring. Such a stance is alien to all that being a good parent implies. To cope effectively with these necessary matters requires fortitude, inner strength, and courage. The extent of these attributes in most parents is admirable, but they should also be fostered through a much more effective alliance with the staff than often exists.

STAFF VERSUS ANXIETY

In preceding pages we have introduced the concept that the need to defend oneself against anxiety is not limited to patients alone. Staff also must contend with the particular set of stresses engendered by the demands of their professions. In average situations experience and training have provided a variety of readily invoked and effective responses, primarily based on intellectualization, denial, and repression. There are, however, circumstances in which such mechanisms are particularly vulnerable and where the professional's usually competent defenses may be threatened or compromised.

Tensions raised in having to deal with the seriously ill, the profoundly handicapped, or the dying are cases in point. Also often encountered are problems in dealing with the "difficult" family and with patients or parents who are demanding, obstructionistic, manipulative, provocative, persistently depressed, or seriously emotionally disturbed. Indeed, we have deemed these issues of sufficient importance to warrant their own special chapters, and we raise them here solely to complete this profile.

No less capable of disrupting normal staff equilibrium are illness, fatigue, or personal problems among professionals themselves. To be preoccupied with one's own difficulties or to be compromised by feeling exhausted or ill obviously restricts the degree to which one can constructively deal with the problems of others. In a similar vein are the limitations and stresses imposed by inexperience or inadequate ward coverage. Here, too, a professional's inner strengths and reserves are strained. In the first instance this is secondary to the anxieties and concerns over being a novice and making a mistake, coupled with the diversion of energies into the search for that practical, easy "know-how" and efficiency that only time and experience can bring. In the second set of circumstances, profound frustration can occur when an overburdened staff member must carry a load well beyond one person's capacity. As work falls further and further behind, professional standards may have to be consciously compromised just to keep up with the barest minimum. Matters are then compounded by guilt arising from the fear of perhaps missing something important as well.

A final situation that is often apt to engender special anxiety arises when one member of the staff creates difficulties for others. He or she may cause dissension in the ranks by assuming an inappropriate role or expecting this of others; by having major problems in interpersonal relationships; by repeatedly failing to carry out assigned tasks; or by continually neglecting to convey essential information to those who need to know. Fortunately, these and other such personnel problems are not all that common. But they do crop up from time to time on every ward and throw the proverbial monkey wrench into the workings of an otherwise smoothly running floor.

STAFF DEFENSE MECHANISMS

Having pointed out that hospital staff members are subject to a variety of specific stresses of their own, let us note that they also resort to various defensive devices to deal with them. Dynamically, these are much the same as those used by patients (chapter 4), although invoked under a different set of provocations. Since coping is a universal experience, we shall not look at all possible combinations and permutations but, rather, shall limit our discussion to those responses that professionals are particularly apt to use and that sometimes create their own set of problems as well.

Intellectualization and Denial.   In combination, these two devices are probably the most commonly employed of all. Here anxiety is managed by viewing the patient in a detached manner as if he or she were a disease or organ system, bereft of the individual personality in whom this is all taking place. Such an approach is particularly characteristic of house staff and, to a variable extent, of attending physicians as well. It is manifested in the long impersonal conversations on ward rounds outside the patient's door, followed by only the most cursory "hello" and "goodbye" to the patient himself. In this way professionals manage to avoid more involving relationships and the concomitant discomfort of identifying with the very one whom they must hurt, or who they know must face an uncertain future. This is perhaps the simplest and most easily invoked method of avoiding interpersonal emotional entanglements, which are seen as interfering with making clear, unbiased, scientifically based judgments.

On one hand, of course, a certain amount of intellectualization and denial is necessary for the sound conduct of medical affairs. On the other hand, their persistent and exclusive use tends to dehumanize, with the consequence of placing major barriers in the way of realizing the full, mutually beneficial potentials of a more open and shared staff-patient relationship.

For the most part, medical and nursing education strongly fosters the intellectual approach as the major coping response to professionally engendered anxiety. Usually, little opportunity is provided for ventilation, self-understanding, and working through. This is regrettable, for a disciplined affective and empathetic approach toward the patient is only possible when one is aware—at least to some extent—of the genesis of one's own inner feelings. Attempting to ignore them leaves tensions smoldering beneath the surface calm, only to erupt in a more deleterious manner at some later date.

Avoidance. An all-too-frequently-invoked method by which professionals deal with stress is not to deal with it at all—through avoidance. This may be in direct physical terms by simply not seeing those patients or parents who prompt uncomfortable feelings as often as one otherwise might. Ot it may be more subtly expressed by visiting frequently but keeping a firm emotional distance and reserve, refusing to be involved in difficult discussions or feelings. Avoidance can be a truly pernicious defense because it totally fails to provide the patient with emotional support and represents an abdication from full professional responsibilities.

Certainly, all staff members utilize avoidance to some degree at one time or another. It is often a first-line defense to a new stress and is not unreasonable if but briefly invoked while regrouping one's inner resources for a more positive relationship. Physicians are particularly susceptible to using avoidance. Psychologically, they bear the greatest sense of guilt and frustration when patients fail to get better and, practically, they have very flexible schedules. With both motivation and opportunity, it is relatively easy for doctors, as visiting members of the staff, simply not to arrive on the floor or to find various excuses to keep from having to go into a "difficult" patient's room. Direct avoidance is less available to nursing staff who must of necessity be in more frequent and prolonged contact with the patient than others. Nor can they easily sidestep determined family members who will readily track them down in even the remotest recesses of the ward. Therefore, nurses who employ avoidance are more likely to use its subtler manifestations.

Except the liaison psychiatrist and the adolescent medical consultant, hospital social workers usually have had the most experience in learning to be aware of their feelings in stressful circumstances and are thus the least likely to succumb to avoidance. Teachers, recreation workers, and other similar resource personnel are less apt to be intimately involved with the seriously ill or with those particular concerns and decisions most likely to precipitate acute staff discomfort. Thus they have less frequent provocation than others for abstaining from contact. But, regardless of which staff member manifests avoidance, it is the least defensible of defenses and has no place in the basic management approach.

Overidentification.   Overidentification with the patient is the opposite side of the coin from avoidance. It tends to occur when events prompt unconscious parallels to the professional's own past. When the patient or his family look, act, or communicate in a manner that reminds the staff member of his own experiences or recapitulates a familiar personal scene, these matters are experienced as though they were being directly relived and he were the patient, or the patient's parents his own. Overidentification is, by definition, a matter involving personal feelings to an excessive degree.

Unconsciously, then, professionals may grossly distort their true roles by becoming their charge's special protector and champion, often gratuitously representing and overstating his views. This quite obviously not only leads to friction with other members of the ward team but also directly disables the overidentifier himself in that he is no longer capable of a constructive, professional approach.

Overidentification is, however, an understandable human tendency, particularly for those going into the caring professions. Indeed, their very choice of vocation may to some degree be unconsciously determined by such an inclination. Novice staff members are particularly prone, not yet experienced enough to avoid seeing stressful matters in highly personalized terms. Further, overidentification in this youthful group is even more likely to occur when teenaged patients are concerned. Recent graduates are barely removed from the stresses of their own adolescence and it is easy for them to relive the feelings of these years.

We do not totally condemn overidentification, as not only is it to some degree unavoidable for many professionals, but also it is not unrelated to the empathetic approach that we espouse. We do, however, urge prompt recognition of distorted and inappropriate patient championship and compassionate assistance for those who have succumbed to it. Once they understand this mechanism, their feelings may be tempered and converted into a more reality-based advocacy.

Frustration and Anger.   No staff member is exempt from occasional feelings of frustration and anger. These may arise consequent to a variety of underlying provocations. In some instances, they may represent projection or displacement, reflecting the professional's own personal sense of inadequacy and failure. This is particularly likely to occur when the patient's condition is unresponsive to even the most vigorous application of medical skills, when the very best of diagnostic efforts fails to reveal the cause of serious symptomatology, or when other such situations occur wherein the staff must deal directly with their own inability to help and experience the repudiation of their very professional purpose.

A second precipitating cause is the patient or parent who either refuses to consent to recommended care or is uncooperative in following the treatment plan. Although the cause of these and other resistant behaviors is deeply rooted in the parent's or patient's inner perception of the patient's plight, professionals often fail to recognize this and tend to see such actions as deliberate affronts to their best efforts. Generally staff members then attempt to deal with the situation manipulatively, first through rational appeal and then via threats relating to the dire physical consequences of noncompliance. When these measures fail, as they often will, particularly with adolescents, frustration and exasperation may ensue. Virtually every professional is occasionally susceptible to anger under these circumstances. But this does not mean that it is an especially effective response. Rather, the resolution of the dilemma will be found in recognizing that no patient consciously wishes to jeopardize his or her health and in attempting to discover the underlying cause of his or her behavior.

CASE 40.   A 14-year-old girl with epilepsy was admitted for exacerbation of previously well-controlled seizures. The formerly effective dose of 300 mgm. of diphenylhydantoin had been doubled without relief of her symptoms. Blood tests in the hospital revealed no presence of the drug at all.

On further questioning, the following picture emerged. The girl was in the midst of emancipation struggles at home. Yet repeatedly throughout the day her mother, father, and an older sister, each in turn, reminded her to take her medication. Although she recognized that she was harming herself, she was nonetheless incapable of acceding to the admonishments of those whose control she was contesting. Thus her problem was not that her condition was deteriorating or that she was just being unreasonably stubborn but, rather, that she was emotionally unable to "do as she was told" because of quite normal development conflicts.

Initially, her doctors scolded her and discharged her after a stern lecture while also advising the parents to redouble their supervisory efforts. Of course her seizures continued. It was only when the real root cause was taken into consideration and the girl's need to control her own fate recognized that the solution was found. The patient was helped to become aware of this self-defeating mechanism, and then was given sole responsibility for taking medication herself, with parents strictly enjoined from saying a word. The girl was further told that if she wanted to control her seizures it was entirely up to her and that no coercion would be used. Thereafter, she regularly took her previously effective dose of medication on her own initiative and her convulsions promptly ceased.

Frustration and anger can also be provoked when the patient or family struggles for control over care. Difficulty is likely both with adolescents, who are seeking autonomy, and their parents, who feel doubly threatened: they find their parental role not only challenged by the emancipation drives of their offspring but yet further "usurped" by health care professionals. Here, nurses tend to be most vulnerable. It can be difficult indeed for them always to keep their "cool" when a teen-ager repeatedly contests such matters as being awakened early in the morning for routine care, eating a meal he does not like, or taking an unpleasant medication; or when parents hover protectively at the bedside around the clock, darting out the door to waylay any passing staff member in search of information, or demanding this, that, and the other for their child.

Last, the professional who is exposed to the stresses of also having to cope with personal problems, fatigue, or overwork is prone to reveal this burden in outward expressions of anger, even where the precipitating cause is minute and would ordinarily be either shrugged off or dealt with in more positive terms.

Of course, hardly a health professional alive has not succumbed to the less felicitous of these foregoing responses at one time or another, and it is safe to say that those who do have such feelings also often experience dismay and confusion at their intensity. A doctor who finds it painfully difficult to visit a seriously disfigured or dying youth does not always appreciate his own inner turmoil; nor does a nurse, frustrated by a teen-ager who refuses to get out of bed and whines endlessly about pain, often view her consequent anger with equanimity. Nonetheless, because these defenses are unconsciously mediated, professionals who are their victims often feel incapable of exerting self-control, and in consequence experience even more distress and enter into an escalating cycle of less-than-helpful responses. It is our proposition, however, that such matters can indeed be resolved and to a large extent avoided through an interdisciplinary team approach wherein responsibilities are shared and feelings and problems openly explored; but there is no answer when each professional works independently of every other and when difficult situations must be borne alone.

STAFF VERSUS ADOLESCENTS

Staff-Adolescent Conflicts.   Up to this point we have dealt with general themes. We turn now to look specifically at those staff-adolescent patient interactions that are unique to this age group and that may pose particular conflicts. For some health professionals simply having to care for teem-agers, in and of itself, is difficult. Few are truly trained and experienced in the health needs of youth and they may find themselves quite perplexed when their young patients do not conform to their own particular set of professional expectancies, usually derived from an education that focuses largely on children or adults.

Matters may be further confused when the staff member's own personal experiences, prejudices, attitudes, or feelings about teen-agers as a class interfere with his or her ability to see the patient objectively as a unique individual in nonjudgmental and empathetic terms. Such may not only be through the process of overidentification, as we have already described, but also through the obverse of rejection and avoidance stemming from stereotyped views and personal biases of adolescents as troublemakers. Further, the teen-ager's common refusal to passively accept the authority of the staff, due to normal emancipation drives, may often be perceived as a direct threat to the professional's own autonomy, with a resultant struggle for control that can end only in mutual hostility and dislike.

Social and personal attitudes toward adolescents today tend to be both polarized and political, wherein youth is seen as either the new hope for liberalism and progress, if one supports these views, or the incarnation of licentiousness, if one is of a more conservative persuasion. Rarely are adolescents viewed in neutral or unbiased terms. And the fact that teen-agers as individuals are as varied in their opinions, beliefs, and practices as are the adults who spawned them is often overlooked. Staff persons inexperienced in working with youth are not singularly less exempt from subscribing to such generalities than is the population at large.

Another problem rests in the aforementioned tendency of hospital personnel to see themselves as benevolent parental figures. The consequence of applying this role to adolescents is only to recapitulate the youth's emancipation conflicts with his own parents. The better alternative, by far, is to become that extraparental adult who is not party to this struggle and to whom the teen-ager can comfortably relate, see as a role model, and turn for support, encouragement, and guidance. All adolescents need and look for such persons outside the family unit and can be greatly benefited by them.

A further difficulty in staff-patient interactions rests in the fact that teen-agers enjoy deliberately setting themselves apart from other age groups in the service of their own individuation. This accounts for the "teen" subculture with its own dress, vocabulary, mannerisms, music, interests, and the like. When young people see their special modes of expression being incorporated into the patterns of others and their individuality compromised, they tend to abandon them promptly and to take up new ways. Thus it may be quite difficult to keep up with youth trends and to be *au courant* with the latest "in" matters. Moreover, hospital staff who attempt to simulate teen-agers in idiom, dress, or style in order to win them over (or to recapture their own youth) are bound to be regarded as both flying false colors and trespassing on the teen-age preserve. In consequence, the pseudo-"hip" professional will be rejected just as effectively as the one who attempts to be a highly conventional parental model. It is indeed a fine art to negotiate that narrow path whereby staff members can come to express themselves in terms that the adolescent can perceive as honest for the professional and that are at the same time responsive and sensitive to the youth's own needs and life style.

Of course, these calculated differences and the adolescent's attempt to take over control and establish himself as an autonomous individual also rouse other anxieties in adults beyond those engendered by communication or generation gaps. For young people are, indeed, unconsciously feared by their elders, whom they threaten to depose and consign to retirement as they rise to become the next generation in charge. We suggest that the motivation of some staff members in trying to control and limit adolescents is not based solely on paternalistic benevolence, but that it also bears a measure of concern for keeping young people in their place lest the professionals' own autonomy and authority be taken from them.

Our final staff-adolescent dynamic consideration is in marked contrast to the foregoing. In chapter 1 we pointed out the conflictual nature of the teen years and their normative confusions, ambivalences, and alternations of mood. For the most part we, as adults, have blocked our own recollections of these painful events and tend to think of our youth as a period of carefree good times. Working closely with teen-agers who are actively experiencing this turmoil, however, tends to reactivate the less happy aspects of one's own adolescence. Obviously this too can be a threatening experience for some staff persons to contend with and can result in an anxious, hesitant, defensive approach.

An optimal relationship is one in which the staff member is knowledgeable about and comfortable in caring for adolescents, enjoys their enthusiasm and vigor, and respects their capacity for responsibility while at the same time recognizing their need for appropriate limits in protecting them from impulsive excesses. It cannot be denied that adolescence is a time of experimentation into the unknown and that young people do need help to keep from harming themselves in this endeavor. In the hospital this approach manifests itself in an attitude that regards the business of getting the patient well as a collaborative and joint venture among all concerned.

From the teen-ager's point of view, staff members may be seen in a variety of ways. Precisely how will be determined by the youth's inner fantasies and preconceptions, by outer reality, or—as is usually the case—by a combination of the two. We have already mentioned the tendency of staff to assume a parental role or that of some other authority figure, and many youths will so regard them. Professionals may also be perceived as symbols or agents of the "establishment," determined to curtail adolescent strivings for independence; or staff may become targets for the projection of anger, guilt, or fear of abandonment. In a more positive way, staff members may constructively be seen as meaningful extraparental adults or ego ideals. Most advantageously, however, this latter view will be combined with one in which health care professionals come to be regarded as concerned and caring adults whom the youth can trust and rely on on order to get well.

Limit Setting.   Those staff attitudes and approaches that reflect distorted fantasies and past prejudices, rather than being based on a clearheaded responsiveness to adolescent developmental needs, inevitably precipitate a number of specific problems. In particular, it may be difficult to set realistic limits if staff function in an authoritarian manner without some willingness to be flexible. Certainly there are appropriate boundaries beyond which the adolescent should not go as determined by the necessities of illness, by the requirements of a group setting, by broader social expectancies, and by the teen-ager's need to be protected from the deleterious consequences of his own experimentation. Thus we by no means advocate total permissiveness. But what limits are established and how they are enforced is important. One can define them quite narrowly and impose them in a rigid and uncompromising manner, with motives of maintaining strict discipline and control, or one can establish a set of somewhat flexible guidelines that will both help the youth get well and prevent chaos on the ward.

In this second view, the youth is invited to share in a cooperative venture, not treated as a pawn whose moves are decided and dictatorily enforced from above. This approach is both developmentally appropriate and pragmatically sound. For it is difficult to enforce rules and regulations or to impose sanctions for their violation upon a physically and intellectually mature youth who sees such acts as dogmatic and irrational. Aside from the fact that we believe an adversarial relationship between young people and adults has no place on the adolescent ward, in such an atmosphere one will either encounter unyielding physical resistance or be outwitted at every turn. Not only is the collaborative, shared approach toward discipline more practical and easily implemented, but it is also usually perceived as responsive, rational, and realistic by the adolescent himself and hence more readily accepted.

However, this is not always the case. Some youths repeatedly transgress such standards, far in excess of a reasonable amount of testing. Such challenges should not be seen as warranting extra disciplinary measures but rather as evidencing symptoms of serious emotional distress and maladaptive coping defenses that should be investigated and resolved. In our experience most adolescent patients do want to live up to the responsibilities expected of them and will try very hard to do so. When they are unable to, this is a sign that they need help, not punishment.

In any event, we firmly commend an approach in which limits are not applied in a contest for control that no one can ever win. This is a fatal step when dealing with this age group, akin to waving a red flag at a bull. Rather, limit setting is simply following commonsense rules by which a group of people can live and work together effectively with the goal of getting the patient well.

CASE 41.   A 14-year-old boy, in traction for a fractured femur, was watching the last minutes of a close football game involving his favorite team. However, it was considerably past the time for lights out on the ward. The nursing supervisor on her rounds berated the charge nurse for her laxity, was unresponsive to the boy's reasoned request to keep the television on until the end of the game, and summarily snapped off the set herself. That the youth became angry and heaved his bedside water carafe at her and subsequently was somewhat hostile and uncooperative on the ward should have been no surprise.

In managing adolescents there is always room for flexibility and rational compromise. Letting an anxious or bored youth keep the television on past usual lights-out hour if it is disturbing no one, delaying a painful treatment a bit to allow the patient control over its timing at least, overlooking a skipped breakfast and a late sleeper, or occasionally omitting the daily bath if so requested, will not be taken as permission for even greater excesses but as humane and empathetic responses. In turn, this approach will generate even better cooperation in the future and minimize struggles over control.

However, one problem about implementing "appropriate" limit-setting measures is that various staff members may have different attitudes and interpretations as to what this really means. If a coordinated and unified approach has not been well worked out in advance, different signals will emanate from different professionals. Thus one person may be quite relaxed about the number of peer visitors on the ward, while another will be much more restrictive. Another example might be the youth who is told he can ambulate freely by one physician yet receives much more cautionary instructions from another. Not only will such situations be confusing to the patient, but staff are also setting themselves up for being manipulated by a bright youth or his family, who will readily pit one professional against another in the service of maintaining their own autonomy. This kind of difficulty is apt to be a particular problem between one nursing shift and another, or when several doctors share responsibility for the same patient.

Institutional Rigidities.   Closely allied to the preceding are the problems posed by institutional rigidities. Few adolescents will perceive the fixed regularity of daily ward routines as having relevance for them. Rarely will they be understanding of or sympathetic to schedules deriving from staff convenience in such matters as bathing, meal times, visiting hours, ward rounds, test procedures, medication dispensing, or lights out.

Hospital schedules also may be strong, unpleasant reminders of contested authoritarian experiences in schools and at home. Further, it is just at this time when the youth, because of his illness, is most intensely and narcissistically preoccupied with his own needs and least inclined to be considerate of the needs of others. Thus, routines and rigidities that subsume concerns for the individual to those of the institutional whole bear very real potentials for precipitating anger and hostility in the youth who feels his own requirements are held as secondary to those of the staff, hospital, or even other patients. Indeed, we suggest that such a response is not entirely unreasonable or unrealistic in some situations and, even though it may be difficult to be flexible in timing various routines to suit each youngster while still managing to get everything done, some degree of compromise is always possible.

Another problem inherent in hospital routines arises from the fact that numerous people are often involved in the performance of routine tasks; coordination breakdowns are therefore frequent. Each person tends to perform his or her function independent of every other, with little sequencing of events. The timing of various events is more often determined by the scheduling needs and availability of the professional than by the needs of the youth himself. This may create particular problems for the newly admitted adolescent or the diagnostic "problem" for whom many procedures have been ordered. In the first instance, the patient who arrives on the floor in the early afternoon may be sequentially examined by one student or physician after another with little pause until way into the night. In the second, the youth's entire day may be taken up with one test after another, interspersed with the examinations of various consultants. Obviously, coordination and planning of procedures to take into account the need of patients for rest and periodic surcease from stressful matters is essential.

Communication Gaps.   The traditional hospital system has no set expectancy that any one staff member bears a responsibility for conveying information to any others who need to know, beyond writing in the chart and order book. Nor are such matters always conveyed regularly and routinely to patients or parents. We have raised this difficulty on a number of occasions already, perhaps even *ad nauseum,* but we consider it such a profound and pervasive problem that we must reemphasize it here.

Communication gaps pose singular problems for teen-agers, who richly fantasize the worst, readily distort what they overhear, and consequently become easily confused and upset when they are not regularly given up-to-date, reality-based information about what is happening and why. It is also important to recognize that many teen-agers find it very difficult to verbalize their thoughts or to ask questions of adults and do not often initiate requests for information on their own. Instead, they remain silent and express their anxiety in more indirect ways.

CASE 42.   A 15-year-old boy with a complex form of congenital heart disease was admitted for surgery. It was planned to create an aortic-pulmonary shunt by grafting a segment of the saphenous vein taken from his leg. Although the youth knew he was to have heart surgery, he was quite unaware that he would also have a second incision in the region of his groin. He was precipitated into acute preoperative panic when the orderly thoroughly and carefully shaved every inch of his body from his neck to his knees. Considering that he did not know the true state of affairs, the fantasies the youth had about how widely he would be cut open can well be imagined. It should have been no surprise when his postoperative course was complicated by an excessive and prolonged period of marked hypochondriasis.

Problems can also arise when the surgeon advises the family of operative plans without telling the staff. So too are difficulties encountered when a doctor tells a youth he can go home but neglects to write the discharge order; when the ward teacher cannot find out how long a particular patient will have to stay even though this information is essential to educational planning; or when the social worker supporting upset parents cannot find out the patient's progress. Indeed, social workers, recreational therapists, and teachers are particularly apt to be sidestepped in the process of information exchange. Of all the problems that get in the way of providing comprehensive care to young people, communication gaps may well head the list.

CONCLUSION

We do not in any way intend to condemn all that goes on on the traditional ward. Indeed, we caution against assuming that because we have highlighted and stressed problems and pitfalls we view all that happens in equally negative terms. Such is far from the case. But it is our purpose to point out those particular points where trouble is most apt to occur and where remediation of usual ward care systems is indicated. The next part of our book is devoted to this end.

two

basic management principles

chapter six
The Hospital Setting

Considerable benefit will accrue to the adolescent patient if physical surroundings reflect the particular concerns of this age group and an appropriate staff is provided to meet its special needs. In hospitalizing a teen-ager, several options are available. Ideally it will be on an adolescent ward where, with certain possible exceptions, young patients can be brought together regardless of their diagnoses or the services to which they are assigned. However, a low adolescent census or space limitations may make this desired goal economically and logistically difficult to achieve. Under such circumstances a feasible alternative is to allocate a few adjoining rooms at one end of a children's or adults' ward, depending upon which service has the greatest interest in assuming this responsibility. To date this has generally been pediatrics, but it need not be exclusively so. In the authors' experience, an arrangement in which adolescents share facilities with younger patients often has its own benefits, as convalescent youths often enjoy helping younger children and thereby regain a feeling of mastery and control and a sense of self-worth. We have found this type of compensatory activity most constructive and therapeutic for all concerned.

Generally, it will be a less felicitous situation if adolescents are placed in adult wards where the proportion of geriatric patients is high. Young people find this depressing and often end up being the errand boys and girls for the elderly. Placing a youngster next to a debilitated, dying, or senile patient should be strenuously avoided. It will invariably increase the teen-ager's anxiety about his or her illness and can often lead to a negative and disturbing experience.

In any event a special area for adolescents can always be allocated in any type of institution, be it but two rooms in a small community hospital, a set of "swing rooms" in a rehabilitation facility, or a full adolescent ward in the larger general hospital. The frequent practice of regarding older teen-agers as adults and younger ones as children, scattering them about on adult and pediatric wards according to their disability or assigned service, with an arbitrary and developmentally inconsistent age division, is to be condemned. And it is firmly recommended that adolescent patients be coalesced into a single area. Otherwise, young people will be isolated one from another with the loss of supportive benefits derived from peer interaction and the denial of those age-oriented medical, nursing, and adjunctive skills that can best help them cope effectively with their illnesses. It is difficult to provide such a milieu under divisive circumstances no matter how well trained, empathetic, and experienced the staff may be.

It is recognized, however, that reality will dictate the admission of certain youths to specific wards on the basis of medical need alone. One cannot always take age into consideration for seriously ill patients needing intensive care, renal dialysis, metabolic studies, or other such highly specialized care. But under these special circumstances careful attention can be given toward placing adolescents in the same room with others of their own approximate age whenever possible as well as arranging for them to participate in adolescent programs such as schooling, recreation, "rap" groups, and the like if they are well enough, even when these are carried on elsewhere in the hospital.

GENERAL PRINCIPLES

Regardless of location, a number of general principles apply to arranging accommodations for adolescent patients. The need to group them has already been noted. Further, except for the seriously ill, dying, or contagious patient, teen-agers do far better with one or more roommates than in a room by themselves. Young people enjoy having their peers about them and are often discomforted by being alone. The hospitalized adolescent often adapts more easily to her or his own disability through sharing the day-to-day experiences of hospitalization with age-mates who are also ill. The resultant tolerance, mutual understanding, and acceptance may not be forthcoming to the same degree from healthy nonhospitalized peers, and the disabled or disfigured youth who returns to his community without this more benevolent exposure to the responses of others may be overwhelmed by the harsher reactions of his normal friends. Additional benefit is afforded through the reassuring example of roommates who have been around a while and have come through their particular crises with flying colors.

Adolescents should also have a recreational area, or day room, of their own when they are up and about. The concerns and interests of teen-agers in television viewing and record and radio listening are notoriously at variance with those of adults or children, as are their differences in other preferred leisure activities. To share recreational facilities with older or younger patients may result either in the imposition of adolescent boisterousness upon those who may find this distressing or, alternatively, in depriving adolescents of activities they enjoy. This is not only inherently unfair all around but also can give rise to power struggles and expressions of overt hostility.

An adolescent day room also provides a wide variety of other therapeutic benefits. Opportunities for peer group interaction and for compensatory activities help allay anxiety, promote restoration of maturational progress, enable aggressive drives for mastery and control to be directed into constructive channels, deter maladaptation, and enhance the use of positive coping mechanisms.

Proper provision for privacy is another essential concern in planning the physical setting. Full bedside screening and curtaining of windows for intimate examinations and procedures are essential. This is often neglected in hospitals in general and is particularly likely to be overlooked when the teen-ager is located on a pediatric floor where staff are accustomed to a more casual approach with younger children. While privacy and dignity are matters to be accorded all patients, the acute embarrassment of a pubertal adolescent on exposure of his or her body to others, often strangers, is greater and more intense than at any other time in life. In addition, such attentions are also frequently perceived as imposing and enforcing an alien dependency and regression. Adolescents are especially vulnerable on both counts and disregard of privacy in this age group may well precipitate panic or some other maladaptive behavior.

Whether adolescents of differing sexes should be accommodated in the same ward has long been a matter of some debate. In establishing new facilities, inexperienced medical staff and administration officials often prefer separate quarters for boys and for girls. However, it is an established fact that sexual encounters among physically ill and convalescent youths in the hospital are rare indeed, even with ample opportunity. They are usually far too preoccupied with the fears engendered by being ill and the business of getting well and going home. Unless the staff ignores obvious premonitory signs and allows the occasional highly seductive patient to act out, few problems arise in accommodating both boys and girls on the same floor with separation of the sexes by room only.

To enforce full sexual segregation has several undesirable consequences. First, it is unnatural in terms of everyday living. Further, it deprives youths, who normally are narcissistically preoccupied with their attractiveness, of the opportunity to discover that they can still be accepted by members of the opposite sex during that critical period of adjustment to disability or disfigurement. Of no less importance, young people will see segregation by sex as antique, Victorian, and invalid for today and an indication of a lack of trust. In turn, this substantially reduces the credibility and perceived sensitivity of the staff and consequently diminishes their effectiveness in supporting and assisting youths to cope with hospitalization and their conditions. Instead, sexual segregation may become an invitation to act out and challenge authority.

Where rooms do not have individual bath and toilet facilities, separate bathrooms have traditionally been provided for males and females. While today this is still socially preferred, the absence of such an arrangement should not be a barrier to the development of an area for adolescents. Proper assurances of privacy are all that is necessary and there is no real reason why a single bathroom cannot serve both boys and girls as it generally does in their homes. Such has been the direct experience of the authors when faced with the need to make this compromise or not to be able to care for teen-agers at all.

Planning a hospital setting for teen-agers should also pay close attention to the vital matter of staff selection. While previous experience with this age group is helpful, it is not mandatory. Optimally, staff should have a liking of, interest in, and sensitivity to the adolescent—coupled with maturity, flexibility, and a willingness to "tune in" to the patient and his anxieties. In-service education programs and experience will render the staff more effective, but only if a fundamental interest in this age group and an ability to relate to them are present at the start. Professionals who do not feel comfortable with teen-agers, who function best under a relatively fixed and predictable set of circumstances, or who need to feel that they are firmly in authority and control at all times may do well in other situations but will do poorly on the adolescent ward. We shall expand our comments on the nature of optimal staff-patient interrelationships in the next chapter.

Close attention is also needed to such matters as rules and regulations, diet and schooling. Rules and regulations should be relevant and meaningful to the situation, meet the genuine medical, emotional, and safety needs of the patient, provide a framework for the staff to carry out their functions, and protect the rights of others. They should not be merely an accumulation of traditions or simply serve convenience if they impede the patient's return to striving for independence. Archaic and artificial controls may promote unnecessary power struggles or diminish staff credibility by obvious irrelevance. Administrative legal barriers deriving from relatively remote possibilities for hospital liability, which impede the development of a responsive milieu for adolescents, should be carefully examined as to whether they can be overcome without imposing undue risk to the hospital.

The dietary indiscretions of teen-agers are legend, but it is always possible to take adolescent likes and dislikes into consideration and stay within the bounds of good nutrition. Otherwise, dull, boring institutional food is often put aside in favor of potato chips, candy bars, and sodas brought by families and friends. The resultant deficiencies are certainly undesirable for a well youth, much less an ill one. Thus nutritionists responsible for meal planning for adolescents are well advised to consult these patients regularly and to take age-oriented and regional and cultural eating habits into firm consideration, medical condition permitting. Teen-agers always welcome hamburgers, hot dogs, pizza, and other such favorites, and their occasional appearance in the daily fare can perk up flagging appetites.

In many hospitals between-meal foods are quite restricted and limited to small snacks of milk, cookies, and crackers at set times of day. The quite different custom of adolescents to eat substantial amounts at irregular intervals in meeting the increased caloric needs of pubertal growth should, however, be taken into consideration. An area with an icebox, hot plate, and toaster that the patients may use at will is desirable. When stocked with such items as peanut butter, cheese, eggs, bread, juices, and milk, such snacks can be dietarily enhancing as well as responsive to teen-aged eating habits that are unlikely to be changed by a sojourn in the hospital. If nutritionally sound and, when combined with regular meals, it meets the youth's total daily food requirements, such snacking can be condemned only on the basis of traditional expectations that human beings should consume the bulk of their food intake in three set meals a day. This assumption is open to challenge.

Last, but by no means least, education should not be ignored. Provision for continued schooling in the hospital for those who are able to participate is essential. This is particularly true for junior and senior high school students for whom a brief period of missed classes can result in their being left markedly behind. To this end special school hours are virtually obligatory. While a separate schoolroom is desirable, almost any space can be temporarily diverted to this purpose during school hours.

AN IDEAL SETTING

We recognize that few hospitals will be able to fulfill all of the following recommendations and that compromises may be necessary. We offer them as guidelines from which to work. Certainly the most desirable goal, fully in keeping with current trends, is to hospitalize teen-aged patients on a ward of their own. Generally this includes patients from approximately 13 through 20 years of age. This can be extended a year or two in either direction, again depending on the total number of beds available, the patient census and the population served.

The precise architectural design will be significantly affected by the existing hospital structure or the overall plans for a new facility; but an ideal plan provides a central core of a nursing station and treatment and service areas with a surrounding U or L of patient rooms allowing optimal supervision and economy of staff movement. The total number of beds allocated will depend upon anticipated needs, but a ward consisting of between fifteen and thirty beds has been found to be economically sound and does not present any unusual discipline problems.

In hospitals where the daily adolescent census is unpredictable and highly variable, it may be desirable to have the adolescent facility contiguous with another area such as an adult or older children's ward. Thus the several adjoining rooms between these two units can be designated as "swing rooms" to be shared and shifted from one ward to the other as the need warrants. Two sets of doors demarcating this area may be differentially opened, depending on which service is using these rooms at any given time.

Rooms.   Adolescents seem to do best with a single roommate. Thus the preponderance of patient space should be devoted to two-bed rooms. Greater flexibility in sex assignments is also possible in these smaller units; however, maximal space utilization and better alternatives in providing age compatibility are provided by larger units and several four-bed rooms may also be included. In addition, one or two single-bed rooms or the use of a two-bed room by a single occupant will be necessary for severely ill or dying adolescents or those in need of isolation. Three-bed rooms are less desirable. Under such circumstances two roommates often pair off together to the exclusion or even exploitation of the third.

For each patient bed area the following equipment is recommended: an adult-size bed with automatic self-adjustable controls; bedside utility stand; usual life support outlets; sufficient appropriately located electrical outlets for both medical apparatus and the patient's diversionary needs such as television and radio; an over-bed tray stand with recessed mirror and storage compartment for personal grooming; locker, closet, or dresser with key; spot beam reading lamp; comfortable chairs for patient and visitor; remote controlled television with earphones; bedside curtains and window curtains; telephone; and a call button or other patient-nursing station communication device. A bright cheery décor will also be welcome, but the dominant, stimulating colors customarily enjoyed by well adolescents should probably be reserved for recreation areas rather than bedrooms, treatment room, or nursing station, where a measure of tranquility will be appreciated by both the patient and the staff.

Obviously, these recommendations are not uniquely applicable to an adolescent ward. Additions to our list of considerations will certainly be thought of by specialists in hospital planning. But two additional planning features are sometimes overlooked. First is the need for adequate space surrounding each bed to accommodate any needed medical apparatus. This is especially necessary for orthopedic patients; frequent inhabitors of the adolescent ward by virtue of the high incidence of both trauma and scoliosis in this age group. Second, doors to bedrooms, recreation areas, schoolrooms, and so on should be wide enough to allow the easy passage of full-sized beds so that nonambulatory patients may be wheeled in and out to participate in various group activities. Other doors to patient access areas such as bath and treatment rooms should accommodate wheelchairs and stretchers.

Bathroom Facilities.   Each room should have its own bathroom with sink, toilet, and tub or shower. Locks that may be opened from the outside by staff in case of an emergency are desirable. Additionally, there should be a central core bathroom with a free-standing tub for assisted baths or special soaks.

Nursing Station.   A centrally located nursing station permits both ease in nursing movements and optimal supervision of the ward. In addition to the usual considerations for this area, particular attention should be given to some arrangement whereby charts, operating room lists, and other written materials that convey patient diagnoses or therapeutic plans can be kept from easy view of the patients. Adolescents are singularly inquisitive about such matters and may obtain confusing and unnecessarily upsetting information by reading technical jargon that they do not fully understand. Attention to proper security for medications, needles, and syringes may also be incidated.

Treatment Room.   This area must accommodate the usual equipment necessary for treatment functions. The only special points in considering adolescents relate to management rather than structure in the need to prepare youths for any procedure and the desirability of advance and dependable scheduling. Procedures that are either precipitously imposed upon a youth or frequently and indefinitely postponed can produce excessive and unnecessary anxiety.

Interviewing and Counseling Rooms.   One or two small offices where doctors or other staff members can talk with youths and parents, singly or together, in quiet and in private are essential. Many of the health concerns and fears of adolescents have high personal or confidential aspects and cannot be talked about comfortably or freely in open ward areas.

Recreation room.   The essential need for a recreational area has already been discussed. It should be somewhat removed from the nursing station and from those rooms that will accommodate very ill patients. Otherwise the associated noise can be disturbing and disrupting at times. However, unless full-time adult supervision is available, regular, tactful patrols by staff members are indicated to assure that matters do not get out of hand when a large number of relatively well adolescents are occupying this space at the same time.

This room should be bright and appealing to adolescent tastes in décor and equipped for a variety of activities. Television will be welcome here, as well as in the bedrooms, for communal viewing. Pool (regular or "bumper") and

Ping-Pong are favorites and provide appropriate levels of physical activity for the convalescent. Double service and space economy can be achieved by placing a folding plywood or composition board Ping-Pong top upon a pool table. This surface can also be reversible and double further as a table for arts and crafts projects, schoolwork, and so on. Quieter games, cards, arts and crafts kits, books and magazines, as well as a juke box or stereo record player are all welcome accessories. Obviously the recreation room should also have adequate and lockable storage areas for these items as well as a sink for cleaning up.

Educational Facilities.   A separate classroom is desirable. This allows for proper equipment with blackboard, chairs, tables, and school supplies and removes the distractions of the recreation room environment. Where this is not feasible, one room can be used for both functions, provided appropriate, quick and easy conversion from one use to the other can be made. The flexible modalities of the ''open classroom'' setting, well met in this type of compromise, require minimal alteration and are suitable for the highly individualized educational needs of hospitalized youth.

Light Cooking Facilities.   Access to facilities in which the patient may prepare simple snacks has been a highly successful and welcome venture on every adolescent ward that has been able to provide it. A small icebox, hot plate, toaster, a few pots, pans, utensils, and a sink are all that is needed. Food supplies should be simple and easy to prepare: peanut butter, jelly, cheese, bread, crackers, cookies, milk, juice, soda, tea, and coffee. The list can be expanded by the additional contributions of friends and relatives.

This area can be a separate Pullman-type kitchenette within the recreation room or in some other convenient location. Barring the availability of a separate area, light cooking facilities can be simply set up in a corner of the recreation room itself. However, they should not be located within the main food service area, which should be out of bounds to patients.

Tidiness tends to pose a major problem. Disposable cups, plates, and eating utensils can simplify this difficulty, and staff and patients together can usually work out solutions if an unholy mess develops. Housekeeping chores should not be cause for eliminating this highly useful and popular facility. Other difficulties may also be encountered with adolescents on restricted diets, who may sometimes sneak forbidden food. However, a youth determined to go against dietary restrictions will always find a way to do so, whether there are cooking facilities or not, and such difficulties are best handled with staff support and understanding in helping the adolescent deal with temptation in preparation for discharge. Simply avoiding the issue by deleting a kitchenette on this basis alone is merely to ignore the issue rather than to deal with it directly. Besides, provision for such patients can easily be made by stocking the larder with celery, carrots, and the like for low-calorie dieters, bland foods such as puddings and ice cream for youths on a low-roughage intake, and so on.

Other Areas.   Space is also needed for other functions common to all wards: storage for medical supplies and equipment, clean and soiled linen, and house-keeping materials; and a food service area for patient meals. No special aspects of these needs pertain to the adolescent.

OPTIMAL STAFF

In this section we seek to define the numbers and types of staff persons required on an adolescent ward. Brief references to job role functions are offered in support of these recommendations, although a more definitive discussion will be found in the next chapter.

Medical.   The medical staffing patterns that obtain on any ward also apply to the adolescent area and consist of interns, residents, senior attending physi-cians, consultants, and private patients' own doctors. Senior attending physi-cians in particular should have had some experience with and be interested in teen-agers. A specialist in adolescent medicine also should be available for con-sultation, to lead periodic rounds, to develop in-service teaching programs for all allied staff, and to share in ward-attending responsibilities.

A liaison psychiatrist is no less essential both for consultation on individual patients and for support and teaching of the staff in the enhancement of their abilities. On the busy adolescent ward this doctor may need to devote about half of his or her time to this project.

Nursing.   Adolescent patients require a great deal of nurses' time, generally more than that needed by other age groups. Time is needed not only for direct nursing procedures but also to prepare youths for what is to come, to support them in times of stress, and to assist them to cope with their illnesses effec-tively. The smooth and efficient running of the ward and the resolution of erupting conflicts, anxieties, maladaptive behavior, and the like rests largely with members of the nursing staff.

The importance of having one or two male nurses on the staff cannot be un-derestimated. Not only do they have an obvious role in carrying out procedures on male patients, but of equal importance is the support and empathy that they can provide adolescent boys. Preferably these men should be registered nurses or, alternatively and less desirably, licensed practical nurses or orderlies. The recent trend of policemen and firemen to enter the nursing profession upon re-tirement from civil service is producing a growing number of such personnel.

A ward will be well staffed during the day shift if there is a head nurse, an assistant head nurse, one registered nurse for every five patients, and one licensed practical nurse for every fifteen patients. The evening and night shifts will generally require one registered nurse per twelve beds and one licensed practical nurse for thirty. The nursing staff should also be assisted by a ward secretary.

Adjunctive Personnel.   A ward social worker from one-quarter to one-half time, depending on the needs of the patient population, is essential. A full-time recreational worker and a full-time secondary school teacher are equally necessary. Last, a consultant dietitian who makes daily rounds with the patients also fills a real need.

Others.   The employment of aides and housekeeping personnel is as for any ward. In their selection, however, it is desirable to take into consideration the same precepts that pertain to other staff. Adolescents are usually affected by everyone they meet in the hospital and do not always discriminate between the moods of nursing and housekeeping staff. Disgruntled aides, porters, or cleaning women may undermine the supportive efforts of others, but sympathetic ones may significantly enhance the work of those directly involved in patient care.

SPECIAL SETTINGS

Sometimes age cannot be taken into account in placement and a hospitalized youth must be separated from other patients. Developmental needs cannot always be the prime determinants of what ward an adolescent will be admitted to. Nonetheless, it is always possible to introduce at least some age-oriented management techniques and to provide certain limited environmental adaptations, no matter where.

The Intensive Care Unit.   By definition, the patient in the intensive care unit is seriously and acutely ill. The main concerns and efforts of the staff are toward saving the patient's life. This is neither the time nor the place to consider other than medical needs in terms of the structural setting. But the dissociative experiences can be profound, and responding to these confusions with reassurance and continued human contact is essential. There is, however, little that differentiates management of an adolescent from that of other age groups.

The Intermediate Care Unit.   As defined here, the intermediate care unit responds to the patient who no longer requires intensive care yet is not ready for the regular ward. In hospitals with large adolescent facilities, one four-bed room can usually be set aside for this purpose. Greater attention to a sick teen-ager's needs can be provided in these circumstances. In hospitals not so well endowed with adolescent beds, the intermediate care unit for teen-agers may be located elsewhere and may include patients of many ages. This arrangement, however, tends to deny the adolescent the attention and support of staff persons who are specifically trained to meet his total needs; and if the regular adolescent ward is able to care for these seriously ill patients properly, they will be better served there than in a mixed facility.

Isolation.   When a teen-aged patient requires isolation, it is best accomplished by placing him on the adolescent ward in a room by himself. He should be as close to the mainstream of teen-age activities as possible. The frustration of normal needs for mobility, peer interaction, and expression of strivings for independence obviously pose severe adaptational stress.

CASE 43.   A 15-year-old girl with hepatitis was isolated in a hospital that used disposable materials under these circumstances. After some days of seeing her sheets, gowns, trays, utensils, and so on regularly consigned to the trash bin she became acutely depressed, withdrawn, and progressively anorexic even though her disease was improving. On drawing her out, the staff discovered that, while she knew it was a "crazy" thought, she had come to feel that maybe she would be thrown out too. Her loneliness and removal from association with others and the attendant feelings of loss of self-esteem and abandonment were obviously symbolized in and promoted by the disposable nature of all that surrounded her.

From a structural point of view, particular efforts toward providing a cheery décor and establishing bridges with the rest of the ward are essential. Glass partitions whose curtains may be opened onto the hallway or a neighboring room will help maintain contact. Closed-circuit television with the recreation and school areas will allow continued participation in these activities and produce a sense of relatedness. The provision of paperback books, magazines, jigsaw puzzles, arts and crafts kits, and so on that the youth may take home or that can be later disposed of will allay boredom and allow for displacement. And, if not provided routinely to all rooms, a telephone for reaching the outside world can be particularly important here.

The Obstetrical and Gynecological Patient.   Regardless of where such patients are located, the same general precepts of support and environment for other youths obtain for the adolescent who is pregnant or who is otherwise the concern of the obstetrical and gynecological service. Indeed, even greater staff sensitivity and tact is needed for the pregnant teen-ager as she comes for either an abortion or a term delivery.

Although girls with reproductive-tract problems are regularly admitted to the adolescent ward, considerable debate exists as to whether the pregnant teen-ager should be placed here or on the obstetrical and gynecological service. Regardless of where the patient is assigned, age-oriented care is essential. In hospitals where there is a special abortion ward, where the preponderance of these procedures are carried out on young women between the ages of 15 and 25, and where a significant proportion of all patients are teen-agers, a highly viable adolescent response system can be developed. The young girl coming for this procedure may be best served here because of the supporting and accepting environment that can be created. The same principles also apply to the adolescent who is admitted for a term delivery. An additional factor in considering placement of the girl who is delivering and keeping her infant is access to the nursery.

There is really no clear-cut, ideal answer in these situations. Both the girl delivering a term infant and planning to place the child for adoption and the girl coming for an abortion are aware that they are not yet ready for parenthood. Obviously, they wish to continue their adolescence and the process of growing up. Such girls will have their needs met best on the adolescent ward. On the other hand, the older adolescent who plans on keeping her child and sees herself functioning as a young adult may be responded to most effectively on the obstetrical ward, where her maternal capacities may be developed by associating with other young women who are also assuming this role.

Although pregnant adolescents have almost always been assigned to obstetrics or gynecology, we challenge the inevitability of this choice and suggest that hospitals should be flexible in providing a number of alternative settings for this group of patients. Fundamental to this decision is the fact that these patients are adolescents who are pregnant and that placement should respond to their developmental status and not to the categorical nature of their medical problem.

CONCLUSION

The environmental requirements of hospitalized adolescents are quite flexible in their application. A responsive setting can be developed in virtually any institution no matter how small or how specialized, and a number of possible alternatives exist. But at all points, certain basic principles must be followed.

1. All teen-aged patients should be placed together in the same area, with segregation of the sexes by room only.
2. Staff must be selected on the basis of their interest in and sensitivity to the youthful patient.
3. Attention to dignity and privacy through the use of proper drapes, gowns and window and bedside screening is essential.
4. Rules and regulations should be flexible and designed to meet the real needs of patients and staff in the ward community.

5. Facilities for recreational and educational activities are essential adjuncts to the processes of convalescence and optimal adjustment to disease.
6. Attention to teen-age eating habits and dietary preferences is an important way of demonstrating to adolescents that the hospital cares about them and is aware of their unique differences.

chapter seven
Optimal Staff Roles and Relationships

It is one thing to point up problems and to suggest ways of remediating them, but it is quite another to put these ideas into operation. We do indeed recognize the inherent difficulties in implementing our optimal view of staff roles and relationships, as it requires a vigilant and continuing effort to work against the strong gravitational forces of tradition and institutionalism. But we do suggest that striving toward the following goals is an important endeavor, as not only will this allow for the best in care to adolescents, but it will also clearly enhance rewards to the staff as well.

STAFF TO PATIENT

Fundamental to effective staff relationships with the teen-aged patient is the concept that all interactions must bear a firm reference to the processes of normal adolescent growth and development. Further, this must be in combination with both an understanding of the impact of illness and hospitalization and an appreciation of those methods, or coping devices, by which we all defend ourselves against stress. Such matters as the meaning of disfigurement to a teenager's narcissistic preoccupation with attractiveness, or the effects of medically required dependency upon strivings for emancipation, and the application of techniques that can help the youth deal with such concerns are at the core of this book.

Working with adolescents also requires a major effort at tolerating and accepting those new and sometimes trying attitudes and ideas emanating from a young person's need to be different. The staff may not, for example, necessarily consider a particular youngster's hair style suitable for themselves, and indeed may even be offended by it; nor may they find it comfortable to work in an area where music discordant to their ears is being played; nor may they agree with a youth's uncompromising and idealistic views on social change. But the professional's own personal preferences cannot be imposed on the patient, and authoritarian efforts at controlling or changing the adolescent's life style to be more in concert with adult preferences will only create mutual alienation. To the contrary, as the teen-ager does have his own rights and needs for individuation, it is desirable for the staff to support the preservation of these aspects of normal teen-aged maturational drives as part of the recovery process, just as much as any other. The business of restoring good health can only be seen to have full meaning if its goal is to improve the quality of life and to enable the youth to return to the processes of his own growing up in the best way she or he can.

Thus the staff's relationship with the patient is one that mixes honest concern and caring with a realistic appraisal of the specific needs of a particular youth. Application of the intellectual approach, well tempered by empathy and a genuine interest in the patient as a person, provides the opportunity for one of the most rewarding aspects of being a health professional. For it is thus that a meaningful interrelationship becomes established in which the patient is provided both essential emotional and physical assistance and support. As far as the adolescent is concerned, we also confess to a vicarious enjoyment of the freshness, vigor, and imagination of the young and their challenges to the old and staid. For this has helped to keep us from being locked into our own antiquity as much as we otherwise might. The professional who comes to be able to respond flexibly to an adolescent's testing and provocations and to understand them comfortably, finds that this not only benefits the patient but also extends well over into his own personal life by enriching and enhancing his vision and his ability to adapt to social change.

It is for these reasons that institutional rigidities have no place on the adolescent ward. This does not by any means imply that one should be totally permissive and take an "anything goes" attitude but, rather, recognizes that there are usually a variety of ways in which a desired goal can be achieved and in which limits can be set in order to secure effective patient compliance. This mandates a constant and unflagging willingness to reevaluate oneself and others in the context of the changing state of the patient's illness and his adaptation to it.

While such an approach may seem forbidding, it need not be so. First, it is essential to recognize that a relationship between an adolescent and an adult does not inevitably have to be confrontational, and that helpful mutual collaboration is quite possible even where a "generation gap" appears to exist. Second, one should always keep in mind that, except in psychopathological and normal transient regressive states, no one wants the adolescent to get better more than the adolescent himself. Given the chance, most youths will try to cooperate as best they can in order to get well. Even though teen-agers may be developmentally prone toward engaging in confrontation power struggles and in efforts at "putting down" adults, this does not mean that these events are inevitable, and that systems of firm and unyielding control must be established. Indeed, such systems serve only to create precisely that autocratic setting in which tension and mutual distrust abound and wherein behavioral difficulties are most apt to occur.

Rather, the key is in recognizing the youth as an equal collaborator in the business of getting well, insofar as his condition and maturational level permit. Many adolescents are quite capable and desirous of such a relationship and rarely assume an attitude of alienation without provocation. This is brought about largely when there are negative feelings and uncompromising rigidities on the part of those about them. To recognize, accept, and respond to the young person's developing capacity for self-determination and interest in responsible behavior, if he or she is but given the requisite knowledge and opportunity, is a cornerstone of effective staff–adolescent-patient relationships.

From this perspective one can establish a set of attitudinal "rules" that will greatly facilitate care, minimize acting-out difficulties, and enhance the more positive and constructive of coping devices:

1. Medical care should be seen as a collaborative venture of the staff, the patient, and the family alike. This requires an open and willing sharing of information and exchange of concerns with the youth directly as well as with parents and other staff.
2. Respect for and acceptance of the youth as an individual with her or his own specific set of capabilities and inherent strengths will go far toward establishing this mutual alliance.
3. Such a view can come about only if there is a firm understanding and acceptance of adolescent developmental processes and the impact of illness and hospitalization thereupon.
4. Confrontations and power struggles over who is in control are to be assiduously avoided. Flexibility and adaptability in the application of rules, regulations, and ward routines will secure far more willing cooperation than the maintenance of rigid discipline in an adversarial situation.
5. However, a definite set of limits should be known by the youth, in advance if possible. This should be relevantly based on the patient's own rights and needs, on the rights and needs of other patients, on the pragmatic requirements of the staff in order to perform their functions, and on those issues relating to group living on the ward.
6. Medical care must always be performed with constant attention to the adolescent's heightened need for privacy and dignity and with awareness of

his intense preoccupation with his body and its integrity. Physical exposure and demeaning manipulations should be approached with the utmost sensitivity to the major threat posed by such invasions.

7. At all points it should always be remembered that, given the opportunity, adolescents are far more capable of rational, reasoned, and responsible behavior than they are generally credited with.

STAFF TO STAFF

As discussed in chapter 5, traditional staff interrelationships tend to promote poor communication in that each member of the ward team carries out her or his functions in relative independence from those of others. In our opinion the resultant malcoordination is one of the greatest barriers to a smoothly running adolescent ward. In the ideal, all staff members must be integrated into a unified whole. To accomplish this goal, there needs to be a clear concept of an interdisciplinary group of individuals with specific roles, whose prime function is to provide care as a single operational unit. We will, as have others before us, call this the "team approach." It is, of course, predicated upon the willingness of all involved to share both information and responsibility under a system that provides the opportunity for such sharing. But, before we define these matters further, two overriding complicating factors should be noted and borne in mind.

The first is that the functions of one staff member may at times overlap those of another. It is thus not always possible to delineate consistently who should do precisely what. But it is important that no confusing duplications of effort occur and that nothing is totally overlooked; the division of labor must be carefully defined in each case. The second problem rests in the fact that some individuals are permanently and indefinitely based on the ward itself; some are based there full time but only for short rotational periods; and yet others are but brief visitors, intermittently crossing the patient's hospital course as time and need warrant. As the ready access of one professional to another for mutual consultation is critical to effective coordination, it becomes just as important to consider how one can develop ties between permanent and transient staff as between the specific disciplines themselves.

Physicians. As we have noted, the medical discipline is a complex one comprised of attending physicians, consultant specialists, fellows, house officers, and medical students. Each hold differing degrees of responsibility depending on their particular levels of expertise or special knowledge. House officers and students are, at least temporarily, full-time members of the ward staff in contrast to the more abbreviated comings and goings of attending doctors, consultants, and their fellows. These relationships are pragmatically determined and reality based and for the most part allow for good medical management and training of new physicians.

But this system does not always afford sufficient coordination and communication between one rotating group of house staff and the next, or between permanent and visiting professionals, or between all of the preceding and the patient himself. As doctors bear the major responsibility for directing medical diagnosis and making treatment decisions, it is essential that the one who is the patient's primary and ongoing physician also assume the obligation for coordinating and integrating all medical plans, including the recommendations of specialist consultants, and for regularly conveying this information to the rest of the ward staff as well. This should be accomplished primarily by personal contact as the written chart is inevitably deficient and too abbreviated to convey the full range and implications of medical thinking.

Further, the primary physician should also regularly and promptly report such matters as test results and their meaning, therapeutic plans, progress, discharge date, possible subsequent limitations, and the like to both the patient and his family in terms that each can understand. This should not be left to others or to chance, with the youth kept in the dark, forced to find out about his medical status from anyone he can manage to latch onto or from whatever he can overhear. We cannot emphasize strongly enough the necessity for the private attending physician or the house officer assigned to the case to keep all concerned constantly up to date on what is happening and why, together with providing the opportunity for all to contribute their own opinions and to ask whatever questions they may have. In this regard we urge doctors to take a problem-oriented approach in which each of the patient's needs is looked at individually and comprehensively along a continuum of the past, present, and future.

The Adolescent Medicine Specialist.   While few hospitals as yet have specialists in the field of adolescent medicine, we strongly advocate such a position. In its absence we recommend at the minimum that one member of the senior medical staff who has an interest in and experience with this age group be designated as responsible for the adolescent ward. Adolescent medicine specialists differ little in their medical function from other primary physicians who limit their practice to a specific age group. It is rather their comprehensive view of a teen-ager's growth and development with an equal concern for the patient's biological, emotional, and social health needs that sets them apart. It is also worth noting that these professionals also view themselves as being no less concerned about health care delivery systems for adolescents, because of the years of medicine's neglect. Thus the purview of this field not only relates to the patient directly but also to the development of positive attitudes and age-oriented approaches on the part of all who provide care for youth. Concern for the effective and integrated application of nursing, social service, and recreational skills is just as important in the minds of adolescent medicine specialists as are the services of physicians.

The role of this individual on the adolescent ward (sometimes in conjunction with his or her lieutenants in the form of adolescent medicine fellows) is to provide general support, guidance, and direction to the staff as a whole in the comprehensive management of teen-aged patients; to bear responsibility for the teaching of adolescent growth and development and related special health needs to others; to serve as the primary inter-disciplinary coordinator; to establish standards of comprehensive adolescent health care and to monitor their application; and to provide individual patient care and consultation when needed, particularly at times of crisis on the ward.

These duties should not be confused with those of the psychiatrist, and it should be kept in mind that adolescent medicine specialists are no less trained in or concerned about the medical and biological needs of youth than they are in the emotional and social aspects. It is true, however, that there may be some overlap with mental health professionals and that the greatest demand for adolescent medicine's skills is most often in the area of sociomedical and behavioral difficulties. Hospitals generally have broad resources in physicians who can skillfully respond to biological disease, but who may be relatively perplexed about the nature of adolescence itself. Thus, while specialists in adolescent medicine consider themselves to be competent in the total care of youth, in many circumstances others tend to feel little need for their assistance in the realm of the organic and only resort to calling them in when a teen-ager acts out impossibly, might be pregnant or using drugs, or is a juvenile delinquent. While these matters are indeed within the scope of this field, they are but a small part of its concerns. We strongly urge expansion of the medical view to include consideration of adolescent medicine specialists' contributions in all aspects of any teen-aged patient's care.

The Liaison Psychiatrist.   Also critical to the effective working of the adolescent ward, the liaison psychiatrist has a number of functions in our optimal approach. There is little question when individual patients exhibit severe and persistent emotional problems. Here the psychiatrist is normally called on to evaluate and manage the particular situation at hand. These are direct consultational actions consistent with traditional roles. The only difficulty in functional definition here is when the role of the social worker, other mental health professionals, or the adolescent medicine specialist overlap, as may happen from time to time. This will be a matter for these individuals to clarify among themselves on precisely who is to do what, and to convey this information to others so that role confusions do not arise.

But, of even greater importance, the liaison psychiatrist is also the leader and coordinator of preventive and therapeutic mental health response systems for both patients and professionals alike. It is this person who assists other members of the team to explore and recognize their own anxieties and maladaptive responses and to counter them effectively. This should be done in the interests of helping the staff to work comfortably with adolescents in general and of supporting and enhancing their capacities to manage difficult teen-agers on their own. In this context, the psychiatrist may lead group and individual staff conferences with the goal of establishing an overall effective mental health milieu from a preventive point of view, as well as developing specific psychotherapeutic programs for those patients who need it. Individual programs are particularly necessary for adolescents facing very serious medical conditions; for patients with premorbid psychological disturbances that may exacerbate on the ward; or when communication breakdowns have led to misunderstanding and inadequate patient preparation with a resultant emotional crisis. In any of these situations the affected youth can be far better managed by a coordinated approach in which all staff members actively participate in the conception and application of sound supportive management principles under the direction of the liaison psychiatrist.

Nursing Roles.   This group consists of the head or charge nurse, floor nurses, licensed practical nurses, aides, and various nursing students. With the exception of students, all of these people are assigned to the ward full time. Usually a quite effective communications system has been worked out among individual members of this discipline, through the captaincy of the head nurse. However, with three shifts a day, seven days a week, formidable efforts are needed to maintain continuity. In particular, those on night and evening shifts may be singularly disabled in that they have no opportunity to relate directly to other professions whose members almost all function during the day. Special attention is needed to keep these staff members informed, as evening is often the time when visitors abound and multiple inquiries about the patient's progress may be made. Further, it is often in the quiet, solitude, and darkness of night when a teen-ager's fantasies grow large and anxieties run rampant. It will be at this time when the reinstitution of reality-based thinking may be most critical and night-shift nurses will be the ones to bear the major responsibility for carrying this out.

Nursing personnel have the primary responsibility for providing direct and ongoing total patient care. This includes attention to bodily needs, support of mental health, and carrying out those doctors' orders that fall within their purview. Although it is not a nursing function to advise patients of medical findings, decisions, or test results, once these matters have been announced by the patient's primary physician, it is their role to reinforce and interpret this material, clarify patient confusions, and prepare the youth emotionally for stressful times ahead. The floor nurse is the one who bears the primary responsibility for helping the adolescent to meet and cope effectively with the anxiety of anticipating surgery, postoperative or traumatic pain, a serious prognosis, residual handicap, and the like. Equally important is the nurse who can calm a restive and worried youth, hear out his anger and frustration at his fate, empathize with his pain, bring him back from regression and withdrawal, and ultimately help him to resume self-determination and self-care.

It is nurses who are most closely and persistently in touch with the patient, both in terms of his day-to-day progress and in terms of his psychological adaptation thereto. Thus they also bear a critical role not only in responding to the patient's fears and concerns but also in bringing these matters to the attention of the other members of the ward team who should know. Nurses are also the ones who usually identify an adolescent's or his family's special need for a social worker, teacher, or recreational therapist; and they are often the first to be aware of indications for the intervention of the adolescent medicine specialist or liaison psychiatrist. Indeed, it is quite clear that nursing is absolutely pivotal to the effective implementation of the roles of all others, and it is most appropriate for this profession to be given the mandate for exerting strong leadership in coordinating all of the individual components of patient care.

While it is neither our purpose nor within our competence to provide extended nursing role definitions, we are grateful to our own nursing staff for pointing out some of these matters and for their exemplary demonstration of one way in which such can be effectively implemented. In this system the head nurse, along with the assistant head nurse, plans and integrates overall ward management and administration. Team leaders, responsible to the head nurse, are next in line and coordinate care for approximately fifteen patients each; but the actual carrying out of specific nursing services is the responsibility of floor nurses in a ratio of one to every five patients. Thus team leaders are free of ongoing patient care so that they can join each physician on his or her rounds for mutual information exchange, support floor nurses wherever help is needed most, and respond to various specific crises on the ward, whether they be medically or emotionally related to the patient or whether they derive from mounting anxiety in the floor nursing staff itself. In this manner a tight system of checks and balances has been evolved in which no one nurse becomes overburdened or remains isolated without the support of others; in which the functions of each is closely integrated with those of every other; and in which effective linkages with and outreach toward other disciplines has been established.

Social Workers.   The social worker also plays a vital and essential role on the ward. Far from being solely that person who assists with financial crises, arranges for postdischarge placement and agency contact, or intervenes in school difficulties, this professional is also a critical force in supporting ward mental health. Social workers are often the primary persons to help families come to grips with serious, acute, or catastrophic illness, support parents of the terminally ill, or work with mothers and fathers who are being difficult. They may also work directly with troubled patients and are often the ones to organize and lead group therapy programs.

More often than not, the expertise of the social worker tends to be enlisted only when a particular problem is identified, rather than as a part of daily routine care. However, it is our opinion that considerable benefit can accrue from having them routinely visit any newly admitted youth and his family, particularly where there is a significant medical crisis. Specific and immediate attention to those arriving as emergencies is also important, as here the life of the family has been precipitously interrupted and many matters may have been left up in the air. In all these instances the social worker can be essential in identifying both emotional and pragmatic needs that might not otherwise come to light. Such services should not be reserved for those with limited incomes but should be available to the affluent as well as the poor, for they are of importance to all patients.

Recreational Therapists.   Developmentally oriented, therapeutic "life" programs for hospitalized children is a new direction that we commend to the adolescent ward as well. We are grateful to the Children's Recreation Department of Bellevue Hospital for so clearly demonstrating how this can be implemented and for providing its singular benefits to our teen-aged patients. In this approach recreational staff members are far more than simply those who divert anxious patients. Rather, they provide the adolescent with a framework that more closely recapitulates his usual activities than does any other hospital event. The significance of this for the resumption of developmental drives upon convalescence is clear. Further, the recreation therapist is quite unrelated to medical necessities and is not involved in imposing pain or invading bodily privacy. Thus, in relating to these professionals, the patient is emotionally removed from the reminders of his plight in a relaxed, open, and more normal atmosphere. In consequence, adolescents feel far freer and less guarded in their relationships here.

In such a milieu, teen-agers may be much more able to ventilate and work through their anxieties, to reaffirm peer group acceptance through social and recreational interaction with other adolescents on the ward; and they may be encouraged to invest constructively in compensatory coping and resumption of mastery and control through achievements in various activity programs. The recreational therapist is the leader in all these matters and often serves as a critical force in helping the youth to adapt effectively to his situation.

From yet another perspective, the recreation therapist is also the patient's advocate. To some degree teen-agers see nurses and physicians as adversaries and as symbols of their deprivations consequent to illness. No such onus is attached to recreation personnel, and it is indeed a common experience for our adolescent patients to confide their deepest fears, frustrations, and concerns to these staff members first. Many youths find it difficult to tell such things to those who are directly responsible for their care and hence more threatening. Moreover, the patient may feel it important not to alienate the medical staff by criticism if he perceives he needs their good will in order to get well. Here the recreational therapist serves as an intermediary and advocate, bringing the teen-ager's concerns and anxieties to the attention of others and representing the patient's views when he feels unable to do this for himself. Indeed, we recommend the attentions of this professional for every adolescent patient as an essential component of preventive mental health care.

Recreational therapy can also play a major role in the specific psychotherapeutic approach devised for an emotionally distressed adolescent. Not only will this be true for those who are unable to verbalize their anxieties and can best profit by working them through via more indirect modes; but this route is also valid for those who are unable to function as before and who need to be assisted to recapture a sense of self-esteem through direct compensatory activities. These are but two of the many instances where recreational therapy may directly contribute to management of the troubled youth.

Teachers.   The major role of adolescents in our society is to prepare themselves for a self-supporting adulthood. This is achieved largely through our system of education; all teen-agers are expected to attend school at least until 16 years of age, as demanded by law, and preferably through high school and college as well. Educational requirements become increasingly demanding as secondary school progresses, and classes missed for even brief periods of time may pose major problems for the adolescent. To catch up after even so much as a two-week absence can be a formidable task for many, and for those who are already academically compromised in particular. Indeed, hospitalizations of even modest durations have, in our experience, often been the final precipitating factor in a struggling youngster's dropping out of school at last.

Thus the critical function of the teacher on the ward is to help a hospitalized youth continue his schooling insofar as he is able, and we firmly recommend the educational involvement of all patients just as soon after admission as their physical condition permits. Optimally, this should be in coordination with the adolescent's usual classwork via liaison with his regular teachers. Further, post-discharge school planning should also be included if this involves such particular requirements as major catching up, making up missed exams, home teaching, a special health class, or less extended school days than before. Probably such matters are most critical for inner-city youths who are often processed through large and not always responsive classes, all too often getting lost in the system. In our experience, a vital need is fulfilled by a teacher who can help these adolescents keep up with their regular classwork, who can even achieve some measure of educational remediation if needed, and who can advocate for them on discharge in order to secure more advantageous academic attentions.

Not only are teaching goals pragmatically directed at helping to keep youngsters in school, but they also comprise part of the ward's therapeutic milieu and the maintenance of mental health through the investment in usual adolescent pursuits as much as is possible. For those patients who like their school experience and see being a student as a major and comfortable part of their present identity and social role, continuing with education while in the hospital can be highly reassuring as well as partly recapitulating a more normal set of life experiences, in the same manner as does recreational therapy. This can be particularly advantageous to the physically handicapped youth, who may need to find his present and future gratification and sense of self-esteem largely through intellectual achievement rather than physical prowess.

The teacher may also become the primary mental health worker for certain adolescents. It is not unusual for some teen-agers to be so overwhelmed by medical circumstances that they are totally unable to deal directly with their feelings. Here the teacher may be an excellent alternative to the social worker or recreational therapist for the teen-aged patient highly invested with educational goals.

Clergy. As we have noted, members of the ministry are not always thought of as being members of the regular ward team. In this day of agnosticism, however, it is important not to forget that religious counseling continues to play a significant role in the lives of many hospitalized adolescents and their parents. Hence the clergy should be actively included in comprehensive planning for such patients. Indeed, in some instances the consent and compliance of the patient or his family will be forthcoming only if the concurrence of a priest, rabbi, or minister has been obtained as well.

THE TEAM APPROACH

Having defined what we view as an optimal set of staff roles, let us attempt to describe how they can be integrated into a coordinated system in which the functions of one are intermeshed with those of the others. This is somewhat analogous to working out a jigsaw puzzle in which each piece, although definable in and of itself as to size and shape, has no meaningful form, but is nonetheless essential and equal to all other pieces in the creation of a complete and unbroken whole. The implementation of such a system is dependent upon the establishment of firm interlocking lines of communication for the dissemination of information among the various staff members themselves and the patient and his family, coupled with a clear understanding and mutual respect for the various roles involved.

Such is the essence of the team approach. Its effectiveness largely depends on certain key individuals assuming leadership in this endeavor. Optimally, we see the adolescent medicine specialist (or the designated attending physician when there is no such professional) as the team "captain." This person serves primarily as a coordinator between visiting and full-time ward personnel—contacting elusive senior consultants, specialists, surgeons, and private physicians—while the adolescent medicine fellow, or the ward senior resident, relates to his or her counterparts in other specialty services.

On the ward itself the head nurse functions as the team "leader" in directing general comprehensive patient care, delegating responsibility for ongoing attention in support of the youth and his family to those under her aegis. She also has special responsibilities for supervising the care of those who are critically ill or dying. In the overall, she works side by side with the team captain in a shared and equal authority. The head nurse is also the one who works most closely with various ward resource personnel, such as the social worker, recreational therapist, teacher, and clergyman, and who forms the main line of communication with technical support professionals, such as technicians, physiotherapists, and nutritionists.

Central to this view is the concept that each staff member bears a primary responsibility to other members of the team that then collectively applies its expertise on behalf of the patient. There is no place here for the tradition of separate intradisciplinary hierarchies wherein each professional sees his or her allegiance as largely resting with members of his or her own kind. This invariably isolates the functions of one from those of the other, with nursing, social service, medicine, and others each proceeding on its own initiative in an unrelated manner. Such parallelism not only places barriers in the way of effective communication and coordination but also promotes firm possibilities for one group to come to feel overburdened and exploited by another. The consequent mutual defensiveness can often result in polarization and politicization between the various disciplines involved, to the detriment of all concerned. Rather, we would realign these professions into a circle of mutual support and sharing that revolves about the patient, its various member components being in ascendancy at differing times depending on the patient's needs of the moment.

Even when optimally developed, the team approach does have certain vulnerabilities that need continuing vigilance. House officers and various types of students present one such problem, because of both their novice status and rotational schedule. It can be difficult to train them while at the same time giving them real responsibility within the team. A major effort is needed to provide them with considerable support in the form of formal conferences as well as individualized guidance. In any event, students, interns, and junior residents do need to be closely monitored until experience has made them comfortable in the comprehensive approach.

A word must also be said about coordination with ward patients who are transiently located elsewhere—in the intensive care unit, recovery room, emergency holding room, isolation area, dialysis unit, and the like. Although essential medical data are usually conveyed readily from one such place to another, information relative to the special circumstances of certain patients should be passed on as well. As these matters are difficult to transmit through the written chart, deliberate efforts are needed to ensure comprehensive verbal communication between the regular ward staff and the staffs of other units in behalf of preparing an anxious youth for the transfer experience, sharing the plans made for one who has an unusual set of concurrent problems, or arranging visits of close and meaningful ward staff members from the old location to the new.

Implementation. Two major components are essential to implementing the team approach: the daily ward rounds and the periodic problem-solving conference. This basic program can, of course, be expanded to include regular conferences, teaching seminars, and individual conferences, depending on the needs of the ward and the nature and resources of the hospital itself.

Daily ward rounds have long been recognized as essential to the carrying out of regular business. Traditionally, they tend to be limited to the assessment of biological matters and are run by and for the house staff (interns and residents) under the aegis of an attending physician. A nursing representative may be present but is usually a listener and not a contributor. Rarely do other professionals attend. Further, rounds are usually conducted at the patient's bedside or in the hallway just outside. While we certainly recognize the need for this type of daily review, we do feel that the format should be different. The customary approach is not conducive to developing an integrated approach, as all concerned can rarely gather around easily and hear what is going on when standing in a busy hallway, or feel comfortable in the presence of the patient to make more than the most restrained and cursory of remarks. Moreover, it is precisely under these circumstances that many adolescent patients often overhear confusing and upsetting matters that they tend to distort and personalize, even if such things are not really about themselves. Teen-agers tend to assume that any group of professionals standing near their doorway or bedside is talking only about them. Further, they are quite unable to discriminate between medical matters relevant to their own case and those teaching exercises consisting of digressions into obscure differential diagnoses, therapeutic possibilities, and other such professionally enjoyable flights of intellectual fancy.

First, we recommend that daily rounds be relocated in a comfortable sit-down setting (far more conducive to an open and relaxed exchange of ideas) and that visiting the patient's bedside be left to the end, when any particular pathology may be seen by all. Second, we suggest that these rounds be led by the adolescent medicine specialist at least once or twice a week. Third, we believe that, insofar as possible, both permanent and visiting members of the ward staff should be present, with each viewing himself as a listener as well as an expert contributor. This includes nursing, recreation, education, social work, and any other discipline closely involved, as well as physicians. Where major decisions must be made about particular patients, rounds should also include the various relevant specialists. The main business here should be the short and shared review of each patient's progress from the perspective of each discipline involved in planning for the day ahead.

The periodic planning conference should be held at least weekly, or more often if needed. Here the primary focus should be on those patients who have complex interdisciplinary needs, present management problems, are acting out or otherwise emotionally upset, or have major illnesses or handicaps to which it will be difficult to adjust.

The same members who participate in daily rounds should be included in the periodic planning conference, but with greater emphasis on also securing the participation of those private and consultant attending doctors and/or subspecialty house staff officers and fellows who are particularly involved with the patient under discussion. In addition, the liaison psychiatrist should always be present and share direction with the adolescent medicine specialist. This setting allows for a much more deailed review of the patient's needs and how these may best be coordinated, together with information exchange and long-range planning while the patient is hospitalized and in preparation for his discharge. This latter point is particularly important. Far too often teen-agers end up going home with little idea of what they may do, when they can return to school, what they may expect in relation to their disease and getting well, what therapeutic regimens they must follow, or when they are to return to be seen again and by whom. Nonprivate patients are often particularly disadvantaged over this point, and there is seemingly a great divide between in-patient and out-patient care with absolutely no sense of continuity. A planning conference in this type of situation absolutely must include professionals from the ambulatory sector as well. If there are problems related to the patient's education, representatives from the youngster's school should also attend.

Such a conference also affords an opportunity for the clarification of mixed communications and confusions, and for the development of a unified approach toward the patient in which each professional knows and understands his role and function in relation to that of every other in a mutually interdependent and cohesive whole. Major problems are created when one staff member duplicates and confuses the efforts of another, or when a variety of different verbal and nonverbal messages are being given to the youth himself. Thus, for example, when one person is highly reassuring as to a favorable outcome (in perhaps unrealistic terms) in a protective effort to spare the youth from being distressed, while at the same time another is more candid and abrupt or, alternatively, completely noncommittal, the patient ends up not knowing whom to believe or what to expect and inevitably latches onto the worst of what he hears and exaggeratedly distorts matters into an unrealistic, confusing, and frightening morass.

This forum must also provide an opportunity for the staff to express their own feelings and to explore methods of contending with them in positive terms. It will be only thus that frustration and anger can be placed into manageable proportions and that the less advantageous defenses of avoidance, overidentification, nonempathetic intellectualization and denial can be ameliorated. The adolescent is indeed highly sensitive to staff anxieties and deeply upset by a distressed professional's own defensiveness and the resultant loss of strength and support. The consequence of allowing staff tensions to fester is to create precisely that setting in which patient isolation, confrontational adolescent-staff power struggles, and interstaff rivalries regarding roles and territorial invasion abound.

The periodic planning conference is also the time and place for working out serious differences of opinion. Divergent views over what type of medical or surgical management should be used, strong disagreements on just how to handle a provocative and difficult youth, or conflicts over just how much to tell a seriously ill teen-ager about his disease are some of the matters that should be resolved here. Double messages should never be visited on the patient, nor should he or she become the proving grounds for intrastaff arguments over care.

Fundamental to the team concept is that no one person can, or should, alone bear responsibility for the patient. Rather, it is an approach that views the adolescent's care as a shared endeavor by a group of professionals, each of whom has a particular set of different but equal skills. Individually applied, each of these skills provides but an incomplete part of the whole, leaving the professional involved unduly and inappropriately burdened in attempting to meet the patient's needs in isolation from and in ignorance of the functions of others. When linked together, team members will form a strong, effective circle of integrated and comprehensive care for the optimal support of the patient and themselves.

chapter eight
Patient Care from Admission to Discharge

Adolescents who can respond to the stresses of illness with an understanding of reality are far better able to cope well with their situation than those who must contend with irrational fears of the unknown. An optimal ward care system aims at helping patients meet the demands of their hospitalization through knowledge and reason rather than through misconception, distortion, and unrelieved anxiety. This can be achieved if all concerned join in a developmentally oriented alliance that includes the patient himself as something more than a passive pawn. Such an approach can both decrease the total incidence of adaptational problems as well as provide for their more effective management when they do occur. For, while it is an ideal goal to have an ever smoothly functioning ward, in reality it is never possible to eliminate all problems for all youths at all times. Panic, outbursts of anger, acting out, depression, regression, and the like are all natural responses to stress, and are bound to occur with some regularity.

TWO BASIC PROPOSITIONS

In beginning to meet this challenge, we hold two matters preeminent. Every effort should be made to observe them throughout the patient's course, insofar as the medical condition permits.

Relatedness to Reality. The first of these propositions is the essential need to regularly provide the youth with reality-based information about just what will happen and what to expect. It is through this knowledge that the patient can best mobilize his own inner strengths and resources to allay anxiety. In pragmatic terms, this means both a thorough initiation into ward routines on admis-

119

sion and regular reports on progress throughout his stay. Further, this information should be given to the youth himself, not relayed through parental intermediaries. This does not mean that mothers and fathers should be kept in the dark—quite to the contrary—but it does recognize that the adolescent has his own particular set of interests separate and apart from those of his parents. Too often staff tend to ignore this point and fail to recognize the teen-ager's independent need and right to know.

The patient should be told, in terms suitable to his age and level of understanding, just what is wrong with him, insofar as is known; what can be done either to clarify the diagnosis or to remediate the condition; and what may be expected from therapy, as well as any other prognostic information that may help him adjust to any possible short- or long-term residuals. When these matters are not entirely predictable, uncertainty need not be hidden, but honestly shared and conveyed within the context of all working together for the best possible outcome. It is also important to give the youth ample opportunity to ask his or her own questions, express fears, and review anything that remains upsetting or unclear.

Of course, when the condition is such that substantial improvement or full recovery is anticipated, it is easy to be totally honest and straightforward. But this becomes a much more difficult matter when the prognosis is poor. Just how and when to tell an adolescent highly distressing news is a critical and individualized matter, best worked out in the problem-solving conference (see chapter 7). While we are committed to openness and honesty with the youth even under serious circumstances, we also hold that revelation of such information must be carefully timed and well tempered by those realistic possibilities for recovery or rehabilitation as exist in fact. No patient should ever be totally divested of hope until it has clearly become a sham and is interfering with his own resolution of his impending death.

It is also appropriate to this section to say a word about the conduct of ward rounds. While we advocate openness with the adolescent about the course of his illness and the conduct of his care, we do not mean that this should include his being privy to rounds themselves. Overhearing their highly technical language, extended intellectual digressions, expressions of uncertainty and concern when a diagnosis is unclear, and differences of opinion over various treatment alternatives only serve to heighten an adolescent's anxieties. He will be bound to misunderstand and misinterpret what he is neither educationally prepared to comprehend nor sufficiently emotionally detached to view dispassionately. Rather, we urge the adoption of a system where bedside rounds are conducted solely for the purpose of checking on the patient and inquiring how he feels. If some sort of orientation of those present at this time is needed, this can be accomplished simply by citing the chief complaint or circumstances surrounding the admission, facts the adolescent already knows. Subsequently, chart reviews, progress reports, and daily management planning can be conducted well away from the patient's hearing. These matters can then be relayed to the youth himself at a later time in a unified and unconfusing way.

Equally germane is the axiom of never taking the patient off guard. To descend on a teen-ager with an unexpected and upsetting procedure may be unconsciously, or even consciously, taken for an aggressive assault rather than helpful ministration. When such misperceptions exists, it is quite possible that the youth will defend himself against attack through combatant or escapist behavior. An adolescent simply does not yet have the maturity to curb these impulses, finding it most difficult to submit to painful and invasive therapies that he neither understands nor has had time to prepare for. Professionals who attempt to carry out threatening procedures without advance warning and explanation have no one to blame but themselves if the youth either aggressively lashes out or retreats in panic.

An Age-Oriented Milieu. Our second proposition is that an adolescent is far better able to adjust and less likely to succumb to irrational behavior when he is in a setting that takes his developmental concerns into proper account. We again iterate the imperative need to be tuned in to the teen-ager's specific fears about forced dependence, diminished mastery and control, bodily invasions, loss of privacy, humiliation and embarrassment, rejection by his peers, physical mutilation, and possible forced alteration of career and life-style hopes and dreams. Adolescents need to be surrounded by a milieu in which they can constantly test out these concerns in immediate, pragmatic, and reality-based terms.

Such a setting provides the youth with ample opportunity for self-determination and self-care to the degree medically possible and, indeed, encourages this out of respect for his drives for independence and need for mastery and control. The recapitulation of adolescent-parent emancipation conflicts and power struggles has absolutely no place on the adolescent ward and is to be assiduously avoided. Whenever feasible, the patient should be offered a reasonable range of options and alternatives from which to choose, and his participation should be sought in making decisions about his care. Rules and regulations should be seen as flexible guides for the specific communal and medical circumstances of the hospital floor and not as rigid impositions for patient control or protective legalistic self-interest.

A teen-ager's narcissistic preoccupations with his body recommend that physical examinations, treatments, and routine care be administered with tact, gentleness, and proper draping. Unnecessarily embarrassing exposure is to be strictly avoided. Moreover, the patient's cooperation should be enlisted at all points. It can be most difficult to coerce an adolescent to accede to a procedure if he elects not to. Far better to spend an extra moment or two in reassuring the youth than to attempt physical force or to bully, shame, or "tranquilize" him into submission.

No less worthy of our attention is the need of adolescents to assure themselves of their continued acceptance by peers. To this end it is important that there be liberal visiting hours for friends from home and active socialization programs among those on the ward if well enough. Young people who have positive experiences in this setting will be far less worried about reintegrating themselves with their peer groups on returning home.

Continuing education and specific recreational programming are also of importance in promoting as much mastery and control as is realistically possible and in supporting the youth's sense of continuity with his customary life style. Here, too, opportunities for exploring and sharing feelings about the hospital experience with others on the ward through "rap" groups, casual conversation, and simple observation can do much to provide each patient with a sense of being neither alone nor the only one to face problems.

ADMISSION

Our concerns here begin with the moment of arrival on the ward—even at the door of the hospital itself. Subject to the nature of the illness, of course, it is most desirable to start by introducing the youth to his new environment and its routines, giving him enough time to assimilate this information and adjust to his surroundings a bit before any procedures are carried out. This is particularly necessary for the adolescent who feels reasonably well and must make the difficult transition from being a "healthy," self-directed, freely moving youth to that of a dependent, confined, and bedded patient. This will be less pressing for the one admitted in pain or physical distress; but here, too, some form of orientation is important at a later time when the patient resumes interest in his environment.

The head nurse or a designate should show the new patient about the ward (or tell him about it if he is not ambulatory); introduce him to the staff; review appropriate routine matters including pertinent rules; and provide him with any practical facts about existing medical and nonmedical facilities that might be of immediate interest. It is also helpful to give him an information booklet for continued reference. If no such guide is available, periodic verbal review of certain details may be needed. Mastering a great deal of new data in a brief period of time is difficult at best and even more so under stressful circumstances.

The mechanics of his immediate surroundings should also be reviewed; how to raise and lower his bed, how to use the call system, the functions of his television, where to put his clothing and possessions, location of the bathroom and telephone, and so on. It should never be assumed either that these details are

self-evident or that a newly admitted adolescent will readily reveal his ignorance if he does not understand.

The patient's physical state and personal preference—rather than simply
custom and convenience—should determine whether he dons hospital wear immediately and hops into bed. This can be a difficult step for teenagers. Some
may wish to remain in their street clothes for a while, even throughout much of
their stay. There is no reason this should not be allowed, except at those times
when street clothes genuinely get in the way of necessary medical care.

The next step is to find out what the patient has been told to expect, and
how he has been prepared for admission. As discussed in chapter 3, these are
important matters in assessing an adolescent's strengths and vulnerabilities and
how he may respond to the stresses at hand. Just who carries out this assessment depends on the systems of the particular ward. Information can be obtained singly or collectively by the nurse, admitting house officer, or ward
social worker, or even be provided in advance by the patient's own physician.

We next recommend that the ward social worker visit each new patient
shortly after he or she arrives. In this way the social worker becomes an ongoing and regular contributor to the ward care team. Otherwise both initial and
subsequent mental health concerns may be overlooked when other more critically ill adolescents, a host of new admissions, or a plethora of ordered
procedures occupy the full attention of medical and nursing staff.

The final step in the admitting phase consists of telling the patient exactly
what comes next. This includes such matters as how many history and physical
exams he will have (and here we make a plea that this be no more than truly
necessary on the first day); what tests will be performed in the near future and
when; and who on the staff will be coming to see him. At this time, any distorted ideas the patient may still have should be straightened out and realigned
with a firm set of reality-based expectations. In concluding, the adolescent
should be asked if he or she has any further questions, if there are any further
matters that the ward staff should know about, or if any special concerns
remain unmet. Again, this informational review falls naturally within the joint
province of nurse, physician, and social worker. Working together, they may
carry it out over the first day, overlapping the history and physical examination.

THE MEDICAL HISTORY

Setting the Stage.   We firmly recommend that both the history and physical
examination be performed in a separate room well away from the possibility of
the patient's being overheard, or viewed in the buff, by parents, assorted visitors, roommates, and uninvolved staff. Not only is it ethically mandatory to respect the confidentiality of health information at all times; but, more pragmatically, considerably fewer facts will be forthcoming from the youth who feels

the whole world is listening in than from the one who recognizes that he is revealing himself to his physician alone.

For these very same reasons, much of the history should be obtained from the patient apart from the parents, unless he or she is unconscious, irrational, or too ill. One possible model is for the physician to introduce himself to both patient and parents and to obtaining from the latter such data as the youth may not be aware of or able to remember. There will be, however, occasions when it is advisable to speak first with the family alone. The physician may wish to find out just how much the patient actually knows about a serious prognosis, or to collect psychosocial information that the mother and father may view as highly confidential for themselves.

Following this introductory period, the physician should diplomatically but firmly ask the parents to please wait outside. It is wise not to give them any option in this matter, such as in asking if they would "like" to go. For it can be difficult to unseat them if this offer is rejected. Simply stating that interviewing and examining the youth alone is a matter of procedural policy, coupled with reassurance that the doctor will speak with the parents later, usually will suffice. If this fails to move them, special problems of overprotection or parent-child symbiosis should be considered. However, some caution should be exercised in coming to this conclusion about families for whom hospitalization is a new and unexpected process, as may often be the case. Here hesitancy may indicate simple unfamiliarity rather than deep-seated psychopathology.

Sometimes parental separation may not be indicated. Early adolescents are often not yet ready to represent themselves in their own health care and may prefer their mothers or fathers to be with them. Youngsters of 12 and 13 years should be directly asked if they would like their families to be present or absent at this time. In another instance, even brief separation can be most distressing if the youth is critically ill. Unless it seems that the parents cannot contain themselves and are about to become unduly upset, they should not be asked to leave.

Purpose of History.   There is little question that a prime goal of the history is to obtain information of importance in treating the chief complaint. But we also consider two other matters of no less value. The first is securing a psychosocial data base. This will be essential in helping the patient cope with both the hospital stay and his course after discharge. In all respects, the history forms the foundation for building comprehensive present and future management plans.

Also of importance is the identification of any other unmet health needs. Few adolescents, other than the chronically ill, are in any form of continuing care, as they were as children. It may have been years since anything more than the most cursory of school or camp examinations. Yet, in our experience, teenagers frequently have other problems or concerns about their health in addition to those that they present. In some instances these previously uncovered complaints may be just as crucial to the patient's overall well-being as those for which she or he was admitted. Not only do such matters relate to the purely biological, but to psychosocial health as well. There are frequent anxieties about bodily normalcy; many tensions express themselves in psychosomatic symptomatology; and some common behaviors, varying from reckless driving to sexual intercourse without contraception, frequently risk serious medical consequences. We contend that it is just as essential to identify these matters and respond to them as it is to treat the primary problem itself.

Obviously, we consider it highly important to obtain a full inventory of all aspects of the patient's health—biological, social, and emotional. But this may not be possible at the beginning of each case. The urgencies presented by patients who arrive acutely ill, or the pressures on time occasioned by a particularly busy ward, often require some short-cutting. Nevertheless, we urge that this inventory not be omitted entirely. Inquiries can always be taken up again at a later and more tranquil time, even some days after the admission itself.

Contents. We shall not examine the entire contents of the usual medical history but, rather, shall limit ourselves to commenting on just those matters that apply specifically to adolescents, or that we deem of importance to review.

Chief complaint. In taking the chief complaint and present illness, it is desirable to obtain separate statements from both the youth and his parents as to just what each believes is the purpose of the admission. Not only may these be divergent, one from the other, but neither may bear much resemblance to the truth. Such confusions do not necessarily mean that the patient or family were ill prepared or misled, and fault should not always fall on the referring physician. Inner turmoil may have blocked out hearing things in full measure. Even when a carefully balanced picture has been given, adolescents are prone to focus on the most dire and dramatic of what they hear, to the exclusion of the more benevolent and mundane. Regardless of their genesis, such misperceptions must always be identified and revised.

Past history. In taking the past history, a full evaluation of pubertal development is essential. This includes the age of onset of genital enlargement in males, breast development in females, and the appearance of pubic hair and the advent of the growth spurt in both. In girls a full menstrual history is indicated as well, covering the age of menarche, the interval between and the duration of menses, the date of the last menstrual period, and any past or present associated problems such as missed periods, menometrorrhagia, dysmenorrhea, or premenstrual difficulties. One should also be alert to the possibilities of venereal disease, past pregnancies, abortions or contraceptive use. Great tact is necessary here and specific inquiries on sexual practices and its consequences are usually best left to subsequent discussions on dating patterns.

This is, however, an appropriate time to inquire about any concerns or worries about physical growth and development. This will be particularly pertinent for those who have definitive abnormalities in this regard or who are at one or the other end of the normal distribution curve. Boys with delayed puberty, small genitalia, gynecomastia, or short stature and girls who view themselves as too tall or under- or over-endowed in breast development or who have irregular menses may frequently be deeply distressed. But even when growth and development approximates the mean, it is a rare teen-ager who is fully satisfied about his or her present height, weight, or state of physical development.

Habits. Nutritional intake, sleep patterns, level of physical fitness and exercise, smoking behavior, alcohol consumption, and drug use comprise the habit inventory. If the adolescent is interviewed in private and is reassured that his confidences will not be divulged even to parents, candid answers in all these areas are usually forthcoming. With the single exception of illicit drug abuse. Adolescents rarely admit these practices to a physician they neither know well nor trust implicitly, unless the medical condition itself is such as to make drug abuse highly suspect or self-evident. It may be best not to press for this information directly; and one can either accept the youth's denial or institute more oblique investigations as to drug abuse patterns in the patient's school and peer group. The patient who states that drugs are easy to procure and commonly used by many of his friends must be assumed to be at greater risk than the one who believes that nothing of this sort is going on. Of course, the questioner must differentiate between casual experimentation and true abuse. Most adolescents will have tried a wide variety of substances, including cigarettes, alcohol, and various licit and illicit drugs. This need engender major concern only when casual experimentation threatens to turn into habituation. We also point to the fact that, in terms of sheer numbers involved, alcohol ingestion and smoking have far more potential for jeopardizing the health of adolescents as a class than illicit drug abuse ever had. We suggest that investigations into early signs of alcohol dependence and efforts to secure abstinence from smoking will be of far greater significance than determining that a youth has smoked a joint or two of marijuana, or popped a pill once in a rare while.

The psychosocial inventory. An evaluation of psychological and social functioning is just as important a tool in evaluating adolescent development as is an assessment of motor, perceptual, and problem attack skills for the younger child. It is here that key information will be found on how the patient tends to respond to stress and where his strengths and weaknesses lie. Thus we urge that this inventory be completed at some point early in the course of hospitalization of every youth. We do recognize, however, that this may be difficult for the admitting intern or resident to complete on her or his own. A number of options exist. The floor or team nurse or social worker can perform this function equally well; but it should always be specifically assigned and not left to chance, lest each staff member think that another has completed the task and it never gets done.

Our specific concerns are how the youth is functioning at home, in school, and among peers. Generally, little resistance to such investigations will be encountered, if they are tactfully handled. Adolescents rarely resent inquiries into their private lives or see them as irrelevant to their medical needs. Indeed, more often they welcome this demonstrated interest in their total selves. Usually, the historian need only verbalize this point to banish any hesitancy, particularly if backed up by reassurances of complete confidentiality.

It is best to begin by discussing school. This area of questioning is least apt to have anxiety-producing ambivalences or to produce sensitive revelations. One specifically wants to know what school the youth attends, his grade and average marks, and those courses he either likes or despises and why. One should also inquire into his ability to get along with teachers and classmates. Impulse-control problems and socialization difficulties may particularly come to the fore in the school setting. However, considerable caution should be taken in ascribing the source of learning or behavioral problems at school to arise from within the youth himself. Some educational systems, especially those of the inner city, are in such a state of turmoil and disarray that it is difficult for any student to perform well. Judgments made in these circumstances can be grossly inaccurate and unfair. Thus, in assessing wherein lies the truth, the examiner must try to determine the conditions prevailing at the patient's particular school.

At this point it is also appropriate to look at vocational goals and to ask what the adolescent expects to do after high school—or, indeed, whether he thinks he will graduate at all. It can also be informative to ask what he hopes to be doing five years from now and what he wants most out of life.

Next in order is an inquiry into the home. Although the composition of the family constellation itself will have been determined earlier in the family history, at this point the questioner should be more concerned about the intrafamily relationships. Some advance reassurance that conflicts with parents are quite normal, and that revealing them is in no way disloyal, may be helpful. Here one wants to know how much emancipation has taken place. This is measured by the degree to which the youth does—or does not—confide in his parents about intimate matters; the extent to which he makes his own decisions; and the intensity of such normal conflicts as accountability, curfew hours, personal grooming, and the like. These are typical focuses for conflict and power struggles in mid-adolescence. Either the total absence of such conflicts or their marked exaggeration should engender concern.

Some adolescents find it difficult to put their feelings about their family into words; and a more directive approach can be used. A simple way of eliciting information is to employ a variant of the three-wish technique by asking the patient to cite three things that he likes about his home life and three things that he would like to see changed. Another useful method is to ask the youth to rate his own family situation in comparison with that of his friends: as better, about the same, or having more problems than most. Certainly, sibling relationships, the physical setting of his home, and family problems outside his own particular relationships are also matters of concern.

Peer interaction is the final area of investigation. Congress with agemates of the same and opposite sexes is critical to the processes of adolescence, and one certainly wants to know if the youth has friends or if he perceives himself to be a "loner" instead. The isolated teen-ager may be headed for adjustment difficulties that will not arise for the one well integrated with his peers. The quality of these friendships is more important than quantity. Some discrimination should be made as to whether these are casual relationships, limited to school, or something more meaningful, incorporating a genuine exchange.

Whether the adolescent has started dating or not is also of importance. Although many subcultural determinants affect the specific nature of dating patterns, at some point during the teen years youngsters must begin to interact with members of the opposite sex. The failure to initiate such behavior may be just as significant as is the opposite extreme.

For youths who are currently dating, or have done so in the past, an evaluation of both the physical and emotional aspects of these relationships is essential. As a significant percentage of teen-aged boys and girls is sexually active today, and as few practice sound methods of birth control, the pragmatic medical conerns raised here are clear. It is quite appropriate to ask directly and straightforwardly if the couple have ever had sexual intercourse together, although perhaps expressed in more colloquial terms. With the previously proffered assurances as to confidentiality and the deep concerns of adolescents about their own sexuality, they frequently welcome the opportunity to talk about these matters if presented in a nonjudgmental and nonpunitive manner. One nearly always gets honest answers if the questioner himself is able to discuss sex in an impartial and open way, looking at the youth's moral concepts and values about such things rather than imposing his own.

Not only should one establish whether treatment for venereal disease or contraception is needed but also the quality of the relationship and whether it is mutually shared, caring, and responsible or exploitative and productive of anxiety. It is not our purpose here to digress into a discussion of sex counseling for teens. But we do wish to emphasize that even though burgeoning sexuality is a critical aspect of adolescent development, it is often totally ignored, particularly in the hospitalized youth whose immediate needs may be far removed from considerations of unwanted parenthood, sexual exploitation, or confusion over moral values. But this too is an important aspect of our comprehensive health concerns.

A brief inquiry into possible homosexual experiences is also relevant to the concerns of psychosexual health. But few topics raise quite so much anxiety in both interviewer and interviewee, and we do not believe that every such encounter needs to be uncovered or recorded, particularly exempting those that represent normal adolescent explorations. We do suggest, however, that the patient always be given the opportunity to raise any special concerns he or she may have in this regard.

It is very true that the psychosocial inventory quite often raises seemingly overwhelming and even insoluble problems. The burden of responding to these matters should never fall on the shoulders of one professional alone. It should be shared through the team approach and the problem-solving conference.

In concluding this section, we wish to review the significant benefits that a comprehensive history brings to patient management. First, such an evaluation best permits a full and valid assessment of any patient's health. Second, normal or deviant adolescent development can be determined in a straightforward and relatively simple way. Next, an understanding of the patient's behavior in the outside world can be predictive of how he will behave on the ward and significantly contributes to planning his care. Fourth is the opportunity to uncover particularly vulnerable areas of functional concern about the effects of the illness itself (e.g., physical or sexual competence). Fifth is the discovery of unrecognized and unmet health problems. And, last, it is through the psychosocial assessment that one can best project just how the illness may affect the patient's future maturation. This is critical for long-range planning and bridging the usually yawning gap between in- and out-patient care.

The History and Parents. We have indicated that much of the medical history should be obtained directly from the patient whenever possible. But there are many instances when information from parents is equally important. Thus the complete history also includes the family's views about the chief complaint, the adolescent's development, other health problems, and any pertinent data about themselves. Here, too, a collaborative approach will be helpful. And, while the doctor is talking with the youth, the social worker or nurse can be conducting a parallel interview with the mother or father.

This is also the time to ask whether the parents have any problems relating to the admission of their child. Middle-class families are no less apt to have financial problems than are poor families. In the face of an expensive hospitalization anyone may well need assistance. There may also be logistical problems about getting to and from the hospital, arranging for someone to stay at home with younger children, notifying other relatives, or any of the numerous concerns contingent to dealing with a crisis. Parents may not volunteer needs of this type, being both too embarrassed to speak of such mundane things and too preoccupied to organize their thoughts along these lines. Thus it is well for the interviewer to speak directly to each point.

THE PHYSICAL EXAMINATION

Once again we stress the need for privacy. During the physical examination, we recommend that the patient be in an examining gown and in a room apart; or, minimally, that bedside curtains be well closed at all times.

Appearance and Bodily Measurements. It is not enough simply to observe that the patient is a "normal adolescent." For puberty spans many years and follows a definite sequence of events. We urge the use of the scale developed by Tanner in his classic anthropometric studies of English youth. It is a widely accepted and standard method of classification in adolescent medicine today. While we refer the reader to Tanner or to the standard texts of Daniel or Gallagher, Heald, and Garell for precise details, we also offer our own adaptation of this scheme in tables 2 and 3 for convenience.

Intellectual and Emotional Functioning. Assessment of the patient's emotional and intellectual function begins at the moment of first contact. How the youth relates to those around him, the appropriateness of his behavior to the situation at hand, the degree to which he is able to give a coherent and logical history and cooperate with the examination, and the type of affect he projects are always perceived at least subliminally, and as such unconsciously make up one's "intuitive" feelings about the patient's psychological state.

   While one can rely upon intuition to some extent, we prefer this to be a more conscious and well-defined procedure, following the lines of the standard mental status examination. To refresh the mind of the reader, this includes the following points: appearance, state of consciousness, behavior, mood or affect, speech, thinking, memory, intelligence, orientation, and judgment. With these as a guide, simple but systematic observations registered in the course of performing the other parts of the history and physical examination will usually suffice. However, a formal mental status examination is indicated when there is any suggestion of a clouded sensorium or otherwise impaired mental faculties, or when possibilities for head trauma, drug psychotoxicity, or febrile delirium exist.

Skin. The ubiquitous nature of acne in adolescence is familiar to all. It is one of the few conditions that is almost exclusively limited to these years. The extent and degree of comedones, cysts, secondary infections, and permanent

ABLE 2. PUBERTAL DEVELOPMENT SCALE, MALES

age	Pubic Hair	Age in Years −2 S.D. +2 S.D. Mean		Penis & Testes	Age in Years −2 S.D. +2 S.D. Mean		Comments
	None; pre-pubertal			Prepubertal; testes approx. 2–2.5 cm. in length			
	Long, lightly pig-mented, downy; at base of penis	11.36 15.62	13.44	Testes defini-tely enlarged; pigmentation and thinning of scrotum; penis beginning to enlarge	9.50 13.76	11.64	Testicular en-largement is earliest sign of puberty and antecedes pubic hair ap-pearance by about 1½ years
	Increased in amount and pig-mentation; curly; still limited to base of penis	11.86 15.98	13.90	Further en-largement of testes and penis, particu-larly in length	10.77 14.93	12.85	Height spurt initiates at about this time; 50% may have downy fa-cial hair at cor-ners, upper lip, and on cheeks in front of ears
	Adult in type; ex-tends about half-way out to inguinal regions	12.20 16.52	14.36	Further en-largement of testes and penis, particu-larly in circum-ference	11.73 15.81	13.77	Axillary hair appears here or in stage 3; facial hair only slightly in-creased but extends across lip; beginning deepening voice; deceler-ation height spurt
	Adult in type, quan-tity, and lateral dis-tribution, extending out to thighs	13.04 17.32	15.18	Adult size, may appear dispro-portionately large in boys who have not yet attained full skeletal growth	12.72 17.12	14.92	Upper lip hair conspicuous; may have sparse chin hair; body hair continues de-veloping well into twenties; growth in height may continue sig-nificantly past stage 5 in some

Source: J. M. Tanner, *Growth at Adolescence,* 2d ed. (Oxford: Blackwell, 1962), and W. Root, "Endocrinology of Puberty," *J Pediatrics* 83:1–19, 1973.

TABLE 3. PUBERTAL DEVELOPMENT SCALE, FEMALES

Stage	Pubic Hair	Age in Years −2 S.D. +2 S.D. Mean	Breasts	Age in Years −2 S.D. +2 S.D. Mean	Comments
1	None; pre-pubertal		Prepubertal; elevation papilla only		
2	Long, lightly pigmented, downy; along labia	9.27 14.11 11.69	Breast bud stage; elevation breast and papilla as small mound and enlargement of areolar diameter	8.95 13.25 11.15	Onset of breas and pubic hai development more or less s multaneous; initiation of height spurt will soon follow
3	Increased in amount and pigmentation; curly; still limited to labia	10.16 14.56 11.69	Breast and areola show further enlargement with no separation of contours	9.97 14.33 12.15	Menarche usually occurs about this tim or 1½ years after onset of breast development; axillary hair first appears here or in stage 5
4	Adult in type; covers mons and extends about halfway out to inguinal regions	10.83 15.07 12.95	Areola and papilla project to form a secondary mound above the level of the breast itself (variable; not always present)	10.81 15.31 13.11	Height spurt begins to decelerate
5	Adult in type, quantity, and lateral distribution; extending out to thighs	12.17 16.65 14.41	Mature with projection of papilla only due to recession of general contour of entire breast	11.85 18.81 15.33	Growth almos complete and most epiphyses closed may grow 1–2 cm. more

Source: J. M. Tanner, *Growth at Adolescence*, 2d ed. (Oxford: Blackwell, 1962), and A. W. Root, "Endocrinology of Puberty," *J Pediatrics* 83:1–19, 1973.

scarring should be noted. Many teen-agers suffer these blemishes in silence, frequently do not reveal their embarrassment and chagrin, and may never have sought aid. Here, too, it is desirable for the examiner to initiate offers of specific help.

Breasts.   An assessment of breast development in girls, again according to the system proposed by Tanner, is indicated, along with the usual palpation for masses. The presence or absence of gynecomastia in males should be noted. When present in a mild form (as most commonly seen), the boy should be reassured about the physiological normalcy of this transient event. It can be distressing indeed for a youth to fear he may be developing female breasts!

Skeleton.   It is easy to pass lightly over the skeletal system, particularly if there are no referable complaints and the patient is flat in bed. But there is a relatively high incidence of scoliosis in these years, primarily among girls at the time of the pubertal growth spurt. Frequently this goes unnoticed until quite advanced. For those in whom it is possible, an examination of the spine should be carried out in both the standing and bending-over position (palms of the hands together and arms extending downward).

Genitalia.   Inspection of male external genitalia should always be carried out, preferably at the end of the examination procedure itself. In the light of our own increasing experience with prostatic hypertrophy in adolescent boys secondary to asymptomatic gonorrhea, we also recommend a routine rectal examination, at least for those who are sexually active.

Pelvic examinations should also be carried out on girls who are sexually active. More debate exists over whether this procedure should be performed in virginal females with no referable symptomatology. However, an assessment of pubic hair development and external genitalia is a simple matter in any girl, best carried out at the end of the examination under proper draping and chaperonage. We recommend this technique be followed by female as well as male physicians when this is a new experience for a particularly shy girl. The formality of the situation and the standby attentions of a nurse can ease her anxiety considerably. Whether one should proceed with a speculum or bimanual examination when the hymen is intact is an individual matter. Although we do not deny that the full pelvic examination is an integral part of a female's total health assessment, we also know this to be a highly emotionally charged procedure for an adolescent girl. Patients of Hispanic background require particularly careful consideration. This culture places high value on hymenal intactness and may consider even the passage of a probe, speculum, or examining finger into the vagina as a moral transgression, with the girl suffering devaluation as a result. Obviously, the decision of when to carry out a pelvic examination requires thought and discrimination. When indicated, it must be performed with the utmost tact, gentleness, and dispatch.

Concluding the History and Physical Examination.   Relevant findings, thoughts, and initial plans should be reviewed at the end of the examination, first with the youth and then with the parents. But, before leaving the bedside or calling the family back in, it is wise to inquire whether the youth has any-thing more on her or his mind and to check on just which pieces of information he or she views as confidential and wishes reserved. Preservation of these con-fidences is critical.

However, we do recognize that under special circumstances confidences sometimes simply cannot be kept, and it is clearly essential for parents to know for the youth's own sake. In such instances, it is usually possible to help the patient come to this realization and accept the necessity, given a little time. One should never unilaterally reveal such matters unless every attempt to se-cure the adolescent's prior consent has been made, and even then this should never be done without first advising the youth of this fact and why.

THE ELECTIVE ADMISSION

Much of what we have said about admission procedures in general applies here in the specific as well. But it may be helpful to inspect what sets the elective admission apart from others. Most notably, the patient is someone who feels well and who is quite capable of functioning normally in a nonhospital setting, yet who voluntarily assumes the role of patient with all its implications for dependency and being ill. The youth in this situation obviously must make a far greater effort to adjust than the one who arrives feeling unwell. Such adoles-cents usually cover their inner tensions quite effectively, but their cool, calm, and collected exteriors often belie the way they really feel. Nonetheless, this façade usually serves them well and should be reinforced by supporting their efforts at self-control and independent function. These adolescents should not be infantilized or immediately subjected to ward authoritarianism. Rather, they should be allowed to continue to direct the situation to whatever degree is con-sistent with their medical welfare, giving them time to adjust at their own pace. Electively admitted adolescents may not want to jump into bed right away and, if in for just diagnostic tests, may elect to be up and about in street clothes throughout much of their hospital stay. In this way they protect themselves from having to deal with dependency conflicts and concern for their bodily in-tegrity to the degree required by being in pajamas or nightgowns. We see no reason why these desires should not be respected.

It is particularly important to respond to the developmental needs of overtly "healthy" youths by encouraging independent and self-reliant behavior and by letting them take the lead. In addition, electively admitted adolescents need far more careful and detailed explanation in preparation for various procedures than others. This group of youngsters can become much more upset over even minor bodily invasions and more narcissistically threatened than those who are truly ill and whose immediate and real needs for care and relief of physical dis-comfort transcend developmental threats.

One last word about elective admissions. All such patients inevitably seem to be admitted at the same time on a Sunday afternoon, when less than full staff is on duty. We plead that there be a staggered schedule instead. It is ridiculous to expect that a reduced staff can ever adequately prepare each youth or take a full history if all arrive at once.

THE SURGICAL PATIENT

Adolescents admitted for surgery experience a somewhat different set of stresses. In this situation the main concern lies in their fears over impending disruption of the body and the pain and disfigurement that this may produce. The staff is usually most sensitive to these matters in patients undergoing major procedures; but they tend to substantially underestimate the degree of distress experienced by youngsters facing lesser operations. Teen-agers admitted for circumcisions, rhinoplasties, herniorrhaphies, or other such "minor" repairs are no less scared and fearful, and the operation is hardly "minor" in their own eyes. This variance should be kept firmly in mind. Any adolescent's worries over impending surgery should be taken seriously, and no one should make light of a young person's seemingly exaggerated concerns.

In preparing adolescents for surgery itself, it is essential that they know the entire sequence of what will happen. This means providing concise information on the scope of preoperative preparation (for example, the parts of the body that will be shaved, enemas, dietary restrictions, and so on) the events surrounding the youth's arrival in the operating room and induction of anesthesia, and precisely how and where he will wake up (for example, his location; what bandages, life-support systems, catheters, casts, traction, and so on will be present; and the degree of pain he may expect). Patients should also be reassured that any tubings, drains, and monitoring machines they may encounter when they wake do not mean that things are "bad" but are simply precautionary and routine measures in their type of case. Patients also want to know who will be present when they regain consciousness, and that the staff will be right there to help. How long they will be in postoperative care facilities, how often parents may visit, and when they can expect to be back on the ward are important pieces of information too. All these data will provide adolescents with sound advance ammunition of benefit in mastering the immediate postsurgical period when it arrives.

It may or may not be advisable to show the adolescent the operating room, recovery room, and intensive care unit in advance. This is an individual matter to be decided upon in each case. Determining factors are whether this will be a useful experience in the cause of reality-based coping, or whether the youth will latch onto and magnify the worst that he sees, promoting exaggerated fears. Strongly intellectualizing or denying patients may benefit by seeing these facilities, but it is probably best to omit this step for diffusely anxious or impulsive adolescents. When in doubt, the youth himself can be asked which he would prefer, and his own wishes taken as a guide.

Another important issue is adequate and properly timed pre-operative medication. Adolescents are at a peak of anxiety at this time and may be prone to panic. The patient must be medicated far enough in advance to arrive in the surgical suite in a well-sedated state. We strongly condemn the practice of deferring medication until the patient is actually called, with inadequate time for it to take effect. If surgery is unexpectedly delayed, medication should be rescheduled accordingly.

Effective sedation and analgesia in the postoperative phase are no less important. Adequate doses should be administered with sufficient frequency to give reasonable relief from pain. Singularly sensitive to physical discomfort, adolescents experience pain in heightened terms. While stoicism may prevail in the face of physical injury on the athletic field or be masked by bravado among one's peers, in the hospital setting the converse is true; and here adolescents often respond with considerable regression and decompensation. Many teenagers recall their pain as the most distressing memory of these events together with the apparent insensitivity and unresponsiveness of the staff to this fact. One need have little fear about the continued use of narcotics and barbiturates for the average adolescent. He will not turn into a juvenile dope addict in consequence. Difficulties with drug dependency are by and large limited to those who in fact have real cause for prolonged and intractable pain, have prior historical evidence of being at risk, or are faced with permanent alteration in a major physical function. An exaggerated preoccupation with pain is age dependent, and in this adolescents are far different from children or adults. Staff should always be aware of this fact and not hold the same expectancies for teen-agers as for other age groups.

Postoperatively, the regular ward staff should visit the patient in the recovery room or intensive care unit from time to time if his stay will be prolonged to any degree. It can be most reassuring for an adolescent to see known and trusted staff members and to be aware that they are still concerned about his welfare and have not abandoned him. More subtly, such visitation also conveys the reassuring expectation that the patient will soon be well enough to return to the regular ward.

Parents should not be ignored at this time, as is sometimes the case. This is especially important when serious or long procedures are to be carried out. At the start, it is beneficial if they are allowed to accompany their youngster to the operating room door. Parents will usually handle this well if encouraged by the staff. A decent feedback system is essential during surgery itself. Hourly reports by a physician or nurse are indicated, and mothers and fathers should not be left alone to imagine the worst. This is both for their own sakes and for that of the patient, so that when they are reunited they need not overreact. Having parents visit the adolescent in the recovery room, even when he is not yet entirely conscious, is useful in reassuring them that he has come through and is indeed alive. Thus when they first see the youth after he is awake, they will already be reassured of his survival and will have sufficiently adjusted to his appearance and state as to be in control of their feelings and able to offer him helpful support and reassurance.

ACUTE ILLNESS

The patient admitted because of an acute condition faces yet another set of circumstances. Here the youth has had little advance warning of what is to come and little opportunity to prepare. The illness or injury that strikes unexpectedly is a true and sudden crisis in the life of the adolescent and his family. The patient arrives on the ward in a state of acute physical distress, often in severe pain and discomfort, and fearing what is happening to his body in most immediate terms. Such patients want and need assistance at once. Preoccupied with their loss of bodily integrity, they are not overly concerned with their whereabouts. If they are concerned at all. The hospital assumes a benevolent role as a source of help and surcease from pain, and is exactly the right place to be.

Managing the medical situation itself has the highest priority. It is patently ridiculous to employ that slower orientational approach suitable for those who are not acutely ill. Nor is this the time to delay matters with a prolonged, comprehensive history and physical examination. Enough time for background details later on when immediate matters are more stable. But it is important from the very start to provide the patient with some form of continuing relatedness to reality. Staff should accompany their biological attentions with a running verbal commentary as to what is going on.

Even when the patient is stuporous or apparently comatose, something of what he hears always gets through. Conversations should not be held solely above, over, and around him as if he were but an inert object, but should also include simple, repetitive, and reassuring statements to the patient himself about what is being done on a moment-to-moment basis. Further, it is best not to conduct technical discussions or to debate treatment alternatives within his hearing, for such talk is particularly subject to distortion by those in a semiconscious state. Insofar as possible, medical and surgical planning should be carried out well away from the bedside.

We have spoken of the need for adequate analgesia in the postoperative state. The same reasoning applies here. Appropriate medication should always be administered just as soon as it is biologically safe.

When the patient arrives in a less than life-or-death state, the early-stage approaches can be somewhat modified. An hour or two often passes before an appendectomy is performed, a comminuted fracture reduced, and the like. An initial period of medical stabilization in such instances is often indicated. And some time may elapse even before the institution of fluids for a diabetic in acidosis or before a transfusion for someone with a hemolytic crisis. While the usual tendency in these situations is for staff to act just as unilaterally as they do when life is in immediate peril, a little time should be taken to explain what will happen and, in response to an adolescent's need to be involved, to give him some opportunity to concur.

It may seem that these recommendations are but a sure formula for inviting rebellion. In our experience, however, quite the converse is true. The teen-ager who perceives that his own concerns are considered and respected and that his drives for autonomy are recognized will usually opt for cooperative compliance, while the one who perceives himself as a victim of the manipulations and impositions of adults acting in collusion against him (a not unusual form of ideation among normal adolescents) may be unable to restrain his anger and resistance or control his feelings of impending panic. A reasonable amount of advance explanation and reassurance—and a little time taken to develop that mutually shared therapeutic alliance we spoke of before—will go a long way toward securing the youth's willing participation in his therapy and toward avoiding those negative and destructive power struggles that are the nemesis of any adolescent ward.

In these crisis situations, the patient and his family may find it difficult to order their thoughts rationally and make decisions right away. They may therefore balk when asked to consent to urgent procedures. Early refusals of this sort are only means of gaining time for rescuing composure and returning to clearheaded thinking. Giving the family a half hour or so in which to collect themselves, while at the same time calmly proffering simple explanations of what is going on, will be far more effective than making a stat call for the psychiatrist or attempting to bulldoze the family into compliance. Nor is it in the resistant adolescent's best interests to knock him out with medication and whisk him away to the operating room unless his life is being threatened in most immediate terms.

Persistent parental recalcitrance is a matter for more careful scrutiny. Some instances will be more easily resolved than others. Sometimes religious and cultural determinants are underlying: the Jehovah's Witness may not permit transfusions, the Catholic may wish the patient to have the last rites of the church, or the orthodox Jew may seek the concurrence of his rabbi. Some parents may simply and quite reasonably wish a second consultation or the opinion of their own family physician in helping them to decide what to do. These are quite straightforward matters, and staff should not let their own religious views or sense of pride stand in the way of bringing others in to help. In the instance of Jehovah's Witnesses, if the adolescent is conscious and mature enough to give an informed consent, the unwillingness of both parent and patient to have transfusions may well have to be respected, as difficult as this may be. If the minor is unconscious, is deemed immature, or has views at variance with those of his family, a court order to procede may be needed. Yet another group of resistant parents are those who are truly emotionally disturbed. This requires a more complex response and the enlistment of all resource persons at hand.

Other issues of importance to families should also be taken up as soon as there is time. With acutely and critically ill patients it is most important that the ward nurse or social worker routinely inquire if parents want arrangements for rooming in (this can be as important for the adolescent as it is for the child), would like a clergyman's support, want other relatives notified, have adequate transportation, or wish help with any other such personal and logistical needs.

CHRONIC ILLNESS

We have already looked at the implications of disease and the meaning of hospitalization for the youth who is chronically ill (chapters 2 and 3). A management program is most dependent upon these matters and the particular set of variables that is operative for the patient at hand.

Acute Exacerbations.   When the admission is for only a few days, in response to an acute exacerbation of a usually stable state, the principles applicable to acute illness and convalescence obtain. This situation is not uncommon in adolescents with asthma, epilepsy, diabetes, and similar diseases that may be subject to periodic, intermittent breakdowns but that are otherwise in good control.

While the hospital course of individuals in this group is often benign, staff should be alert to possible depression or overcompensation. Hospitalization may well underscore the patient's basic illness and activate a new set of maladaptive responses. Where such seems to be the case, verbal exploration of these matters in some depth can help the youth understand the basis of his actions and deal with his feelings in more appropriate terms.

For those who are but infrequently admitted, hospitalization can be put to advantage as an occasion for examining the patient's adaptation to his condition in general, and whether he has integrated it into his personality reasonably well or uses it for continued dependence, forced attentions from his parents, or other such secondary gains. In this context, admission provides a useful opportunity to review the adolescent's maturational needs. All too often, once a chronic condition is diagnosed and the initial evaluation complete, little further attention is given to psychosocial matters in the relative brevity of followup care. Concern for emotional and vocational issues tends to be arrested at an early stage. This can be particularly damaging when the onset of illness was in childhood and the patient's progression into adolescence is overlooked. The deplorable result is that all the unique needs of these years are ignored. The concerns of a youth about his career and adult life functioning may quite escape the mind of the clinic staff or private physician who began caring for him when he was three; nor may the fears about sexual integrity of a teen-ager who is disabled in any way be recognized by those who knew him initially in a prepubertal state.

We have also found long-standing special school placements, as in a health class, frequently to be still in force, although long outdated insofar as there is real need; and early restrictions on activity may never have been lifted, even though no longer required. Commonly, one will also find parents who are still administering medication or other ongoing care to their offspring far past the time when he should be doing this for himself. All of these matters should be periodically reviewed in depth. The occasion of hospitalization is an effective time for this and for revision of his course.

Diagnostic Evaluation.   Another category is comprised of youths who feel relatively normal, who function well, and who are admitted for a special or periodic evaluation. This can be for such procedures as cardiac catheterization, renal biopsy, or endocrine or metabolic studies. In essence, these youngsters are managed as elective admissions (for in fact that is what they are), with the added recognition that they will be singularly anxious about test procedures and results. Particular attention is needed in preparing these patients for what is to come, including showing them the medical facilities, such as the catheterization laboratory or metabolic ward, in advance. Further, one should be sure to inform the youth about the results of the tests just as soon as they are known.

Special Therapies.   A third group consists of those who are repeatedly admitted for special therapies such as renal dialysis, treatment for malignancy, transfusions for chronic anemias, multilple-stage plastic repairs, and so on. These are all adolescents whose diseases are ever with them to a greater or lesser degree, and who have few moments in life when they can successfully put their health problems aside. Here the patient's individual response will dictate his management needs. Those who view the hospital as a haven of safety and see the staff as old and trusted friends will pose few problems. Generally, hospitalization is an easy, collaborative time for all concerned. Of course, this point does stress the need for continuity in care from one admission to the next. And every effort should be made to see that these youngsters are cared for by the same personnel each time.

However, adolescents who perceive their hospitalization as a sign of deterioration, a reminder of the poor hand that life has dealt them, often bring all their anger, resentment, and bitterness with them. In these circumstances, acting out or serious depression are common and can present a genuine challenge. Certainly this is the time for the frequent invocation of the problem-solving conference; and the consultant in adolescent medicine or the liaison psychiatrist can be critical supports. In essence, the management plan attempts to engage the adolescent in as many normal developmental pursuits as is possible through recreational, vocational, and social planning while at the same time instituting supportive or interpretive psychotherapy, depending on the patient's capacity for insight. Work with the family will also be useful in helping them to support these maturational goals, rather than perpetuating the same overprotective or rejecting attitudes that they may have held in the past. In all these measures, the leadership of the permanent ward care team vests largely in the social worker.

Deterioration.   A last group consists of patients whose admission signals true deterioration, as in those with cardiac failure, renal decompensation, malignant metastases, unremitting ulcerative colitis, and the like. This is invariably a time of discouragement, disappointment, and depression for all concerned; no less so for the staff than for the patient and his family. Staff distress may be particularly great if this is a youth they have known and cared for over many months or years. Here, too, management principles are highly individualized and somewhere between those defined in the preceding category and those set forth for the dying adolescent. Of course, much depends on what can be expected from medical care and the prognosis; whether there is hope or whether the admission truly signals the beginning of the end. In any event the youth, his family, and the staff all need frequent and ample opportunity to express their feelings, sharing the burden and pain, giving and receiving support, one to the other. At this time profound fears and concerns are appropriate and should not be denied or repressed in a stoic and futile endeavor to pretend that all is, or soon will become, well.

Coordination of Care.   Coordination and integration of all professionals caring for the chronically ill adolescent is singularly important. In particularly complex situations, many people from a wide variety of specialties and technical disciplines will be involved. It is essential that each one knows what the others are doing and that the youth be presented with a unified therapeutic plan. Leaving these matters to the customary fragmented approach only compounds confusion and fear.

A further obligation of those who care for the chronically ill youth in the hospital is to coordinate their functions with those who manage his condition when he is at home. Adolescents receiving ambulatory treatment in a clinic are particularly subject to profound discontinuity in care at the interface between in- and out-patient services. This is, of course, less likely to occur when the patient is under the aegis of a private physician, unless multiple specialists and generalists are involved. We urge that the ward staff assure themselves that appropriate professionals in the ambulatory sector are promptly notified of the youth's arrival and are advised of his course throughout his stay. Further, clinic personnel should be encouraged not only to visit the patient on the ward but to actively participate in in-hospital planning conferences as well.

Behavioral Problems.   It should always be recognized that chronic illness in adolescence always is in direct opposition to developmental drives and heightens even further the usual preoccupations with physical maturation and normalcy. It is most understandable, then, when we point out that these adolescents are particularly prone to behavioral problems. Compensatory acting out, use of the condition for secondary manipulative gain, excessive dependence on parents with symbiotic relationships, and chronic depression are frequently seen. Not only does the staff need to be alert to such difficulties, but they should also institute specific programs for countering them with the goals of encouraging the adolescent to assume responsibility for his own care, to socialize with his peers on the ward, to verbalize his specific concerns, and to find ways he can gain a sense of accomplishment, self-esteem, and autonomy. At heart is the adolescent's need to be reassured that he is not devalued, cast out, or so different or so strange as to be unworthy of friendship and love.

These youngsters may do particularly well as junior volunteers after discharge, helping out on the wards or elsewhere in the hospital. The teen-ager who can convert concern for himself into concern for others, and who can put his usually considerable hospital expertise as a patient into the service of others, comes to gain a new sense of self-worth, mastery, and control in a situation in which he feels relatively safe. This can often function as a highly beneficial transitional state for those who are somewhat unsure of holding their own in the outside world. And successes here can be translated into a less protected situation at a later time.

CONVALESCENCE

At some point in the stay of every hospitalized adolescent, he or she becomes a convalescent. This is the time when the medical course is stabilized and the patient begins to move back toward health. The primary management goals are to help the youth resume independent functioning in accord with his maturational drives. But sometimes matters are less simple than they might at first appear.

Early Convalescence.   During the earliest days of improvement, how the staff perceives the patient and how the patient feels about himself are often markedly different. When the condition itself no longer represents an immediate biological threat, all concerned are released from their earlier intense preoccupations with moment-to-moment survival. The staff now have the option of removing their attentions to another who may need them more, but the adolescent now begins to experience the full dimensions of the physical insult itself. He becomes preoccupied with his lack of physical integrity. Pain and somatic discomforts become heightened, magnified, and increasingly real. Emotional and physical exhaustion often result in a period of regression and depression until inner adaptive forces have had sufficient time to regroup themselves.

All in all, it is quite safe to say that in the early convalescent phase the patient may feel at his worst. In consequence, staff expectations may far exceed what the adolescent can in fact do, and their demands for his ambulation or decrease in his analgesia may be beyond what he is actually capable of handling. In addition, the tendency of ward doctors and nurses to turn their attention elsewhere at this time may only aggravate the patient's sense of depression and fears of abandonment just at the time when he feels he needs help the most.

These discrepancies should be recognized and dealt with, not only in response to the adolescent's immediate plight but also in aid of averting possibilities for inappropriate staff anger when the youth does not live up to their demands. Instead, matters should be advanced relatively slowly at this time, letting the youth take the lead himself in informing the staff when he is ready to move on. It is highly unlikely that a formerly vigorous and active adolescent will succumb to a life of chronic invalidism if he or she is not propelled up and out of bed into instantaneous, total self-care at this time. In this connection, we again call attention to the very real need of teen-agers to be cared for by those who are well versed in their needs, not by special duty personnel unfamiliar with hospitalized youth.

The concerns of the patient being transferred from the intensive care unit back to the ward deserve particular notice. This adolescent may be highly fearful of diminished attentions, anxious about having to adjust to a new location, and in need of frequent reassuring contact with the ward staff. Even if not precisely medically indicated, hourly stops by the bedside to inquire whether all is going well are advisable during the first day, as are extended visiting hours for parents who can serve as advocates in time of need.

Thus in this early phase we wish to point up the significant difference between physical and perceptual convalescence. Recognition and acceptance of the adolescent's continued regression for a few more days, of his persistent preoccupation with pain and need for adequate analgesia (so very different from the course of younger children), and of the fact that he does not usually consider himself to be nearly so well as do the staff, will all go a long way toward smoothing the convalescent's course.

Mid-Convalescence. This period can be said to have begun when the adolescent starts to feel better. His views of his state now approximate those of the staff. Individual personality variants and the extent of the physical insult itself will collectively determine just how long this will take and whether mid-convalescence will be quickly reached or more tentatively begun. Such matters cannot be forced.

Most adolescents will signal this new phase on their own, although usually in behavioral rather than verbal terms. The tipoff that the patient has entered mid-convalescence is when he or she begins to show interest in television, magazines, puzzles, and the like; wants to call his friends on the telephone; and starts complaining about the food. Obviously, it is a highly useful management technique to surround the early convalescent with these stimuli; he will respond to them when he is ready.

Mid-convalescence is the time when the full panoply of the age-oriented milieu is brought to bear, with the goal of helping adolescent patients reassert their drives for independence, rescue their sense of self-esteem, reestablish their body image and sense of attractiveness, reengage in interacting with their peers, and recoup any educational loss. Optimally, this is also the time when teen-aged patients begin to find a new sense of pride, accomplishment, and self-reliance in having coped with a difficult situation. Scars and disfigurements (if they are not excessively obvious or uglifying) can come to be seen as badges of honor and courage rather than as marks of shame. Management supports these views by offering positive reinforcement as to how well the patient has done. This should be true for "minor" as well as "major" conditions, for such differentiation may exist only in the minds of the staff; most adolescents consider hospitalization for any condition as a major event.

At this point, the recreational or occupational therapist and the ward teacher vigorously enter the scene. Particular attention should be given to encouraging self-care, ambulation, and socialization with others on the ward, to resumption of schooling, to participation in structured recreational activities, to "rap" groups, and to other measures aimed at assisting in the resolution of persistent anxieties and restoring functional adaptation.

Special concern is needed for those with residual disfigurements, handicaps, or other physical limitations. Indeed, special programs for this group to explore their feelings, share experiences, build their own peer group, and invoke constructive compensatory modes for what they have lost is vital. The patient is only partially benefited if his physical health is restored but his mental health is neglected. Once made well again, he may become an emotional recluse.

Of course, the management team's goals may be limited by reality. An adolescent who must face severe permanent motor loss, grossly disfiguring scars, major curtailments in permissible activities, or flagrant disruption of normal physiological pathways does have to make profound concessions in his present and future life style. Working through such changes is a true mourning process, and it takes time. But we hold that our general management principles obtain here as well and that for all adolescents the goal of mid-convalescence is to reengage in normal life pursuits to the fullest possible degree.

There are, however, always some adolescents who fail to resume normal maturation. Patients who persist in regression, depression, or withdrawal are often those who have had similar problems in the past or those who now have a valid, reality-based reason, such as having to face a life of quadriplegia or the loss of a limb. In the first set of circumstances the staff should have been aware of these possibilities right from the start, if an adequate history was obtained. And, in the second, they should be self-evident in the nature of the condition itself. Advance recognition of probable difficulties allows the staff to prepare for them with reason and understanding and not to be taken off guard when they do arise. Under these terms one can be much more empathetic and calm in dealing with "problem" patients than when one has no such expectancies in mind.

We again commend the problem-solving conference for managing these particularly difficult situations and planning the team approach. In all cases the first step lies in accepting and understanding exactly where the youth is "at" in a nonjudgmental and nonpunitive way, slowly encouraging him to move forward along a more constructive path. Often this depends on the close and continued work of one team member whom the youth particularly likes and trusts, in conjunction with the support of the others. Usually this will be the social worker, liaison psychiatrist, or adolescent consultant or fellow. But the nurse, recreation worker, and the teacher are no less capable of fullfilling this role.

Late Convalescence.   This is the period when recovery is secure and medical attentions from a professional staff on a continuing basis are no longer necessary. The patient is well on the way to normal health, except for easy fatiguability and adaptation to any permanent residuals. He or she is usually discharged at the advent of this stage, and the work of the ward staff is nearly done. The final task of ward management is to prepare a smooth transition in handing care over to those on the "outside," assuring that any continuing therapeutic requirements will be met and that established plans for the patient's return to full function will be carried out. The youth and his family must not depart without knowing what medications he should take and when; what special care measures he should observe; when he should return to see his doctor; how long he need stay in bed, if at all; when he may return to school; when he may resume full activity, including sports; and any indicated instructions on special signs or symptoms to watch for and what to do if they occur.

In addition, the patient's course to date and prospects for his future should be carefully reviewed with both the adolescent and his family, and each independently given an opportunity to ask any final questions or express concerns. More than at any other stage of hospitalization, the adolescent will be tuned in to reality and able to understand clearly what is being said. But he is likely to have two major anxieties about returning home: whether he is yet ready to relinquish the hospital's protection and whether he will still have the same relationship with his peers and his school as before. At this point parents and close friends take over from the staff in offering reassurance on both counts.

CONCLUSION

One cannot develop a "cookbook approach" or "laundry-list guide" to the management of the adolescent patient. There are no infallible recipes or check-lists that guarantee success. It is difficult even to attempt a general description of an effective approach. As we have tried to convey, this must be based on empathetic, affective principles rather than on a set of measurable but emotionally distant cognitive skills. Thus there is much latitude in procedure but virtually none insofar as the underlying motivation is concerned. Even the most elegant ward and elaborate program will be doomed to fail if the staff view adolescents in alien, mistrusting, and less-than-honest terms or use the patient's dependence in the service of their own needs for power and control. On the other hand, teen-agers will tolerate even major deficiencies in the physical plant, shortages in staff, and considerable personal discomfort and deprivation if they sense that those who care for them do so out of genuine concern, commitment, understanding, and respect.

three

special challenges

chapter nine

Common Behavioral Problems

From the perspective of health care professionals, an adolescent is a behavioral problem if he or she makes more than customary "waves" on the ward, threatens the carrying out of staff functions, or excessively disrupts established routines. But seeing matters only through the eyes of the beholder tends to exculpate staff complicity and to overlook the underlying cause. By ignoring dynamic considerations, we inevitably become trapped into contending with disruptive adolescents through the stepwise progression of cajoling, bargaining, threatening, and coercion. Too often this results only in mutual frustration, anger, and dislike.

Instead, we shall look at behavioral problems from the perspective of the patient. In this view, aberrant behavior is not the primary issue but, rather, is symptomatic of the adolescent's inner distress. And teen-agers who quietly retreat into self-imposed isolation are no less behavior problems than those who obnoxiously act out. Thus, behavioral problems may be either "inwardly" or "outwardly" directed, and neither can be ignored.

In further setting the ground rules for this chapter, we shall not include those challenging acts characteristic of adolescent development. While these normal behaviors can pose problems at times, they are to be expected and even welcomed as indicators of adaptive coping. We would not, for example, consider a certain amount of rebelliousness over rules and regulations to be a "behavior problem." Nor would we see anger, denial, or depression as out of line when justified by a seriously ill patient's first awareness of his or her true state. These are valid initial defenses that generally work themselves through with time. Indeed, failing to meet serious stress in these ways may be a problem in itself.

CASE 44.   A 17-year-old male had developed a malignancy of his left knee some two years before. As the tumor was found to be both well differentiated and localized, he had been treated by resection rather than amputation. This was carried out by wide removal of the involved bone from mid-thigh to mid-calf. Structural stability was restored via the insertion of a metal rod. Although this resulted in a fixed and immobile knee, the youth did retain his extremity and was able to get about with only a modest limp. During his entire first hospitalization he had been the model of intellectualizing rationality. He complied happily with every management detail and was unendingly in good spirits. He was the ward darling; never complaining, regressing, or angry; never posing that difficult question of whether he would live or die, even though he knew his diagnosis and what it implied.

On return to school, he compensated for his lost (and highly prized) athletic prowess by being both a student leader and bon vivant. He remained free of his disease. All were most pleased with his course and gave little thought to increasing sleep difficulties, somewhat slipping grades, and a certain intensity in his usual mood.

The youth was now admitted for a minor revision of the stabilizing rod because of some local pain. Two days after this relatively minor operation he most unexpectedly became highly agitated, bordering on panic. When finally calmed, a profound depression ensued that verged on the suicidal. He stated that he simply couldn't stand being crippled and was sure he would die as well. At no point over the preceding two years had he dealt with his condition in other than denying terms.

We believe that his initial denial was the true problem and not his later panic and depression during the second hospitalization, with all its reminders of the first. One suspects that if he had been helped to mourn his loss of function in the beginning and to speak openly about his fears for the future, as painful as this may have been, he might not have succumbed to this defensive collapse.

It is also helpful to keep in mind that maladaptive behaviors serve a real psychic purpose in dealing with anxiety, just as do more constructive modes. While some may view uncooperative teen-agers as difficult, stubborn, and "ornery" simply for the pleasure of it, this is usually far from the case. In our experience, most adolescent patients try to cooperate as best they can. Even when a youth has exhibited the most delinquent of behaviors on the outside, his attitudes toward adults and authority often change dramatically when his own physical integrity is at stake. The patient who maladapts in the hospital is truly disabled and incapable of mustering a more constructive response; the threats posed by either inner fantasy or outer reality are more than he can contend with successfully. Whether a teen-ager withdraws and isolates himself, acts out aggressively, is regressed and demanding, or displays other difficult behaviors, this is still the best he can do.

For some patients, maladaptive coping has been a lifelong pattern. For others, this will be a new manifestation consequent to the overwhelming aspects of illness and hospitalization. We have frequently spoken of the intensity of narcissistic concerns among adolescents, their difficulty in achieving insightful acceptance of physical disability, and their singular vulnerability for overreacting to biological harm.

Any patient's basic and deepest fears about his disease stem from his diminished sense of self-esteem and its portent for personal devaluation, rejection, and ultimate abandonment. This is, of course, an intolerable prospect. In defending against these feelings, emotional energy is directed toward either securing reassuring attention at any cost or withdrawing and isolating oneself from having to face these issues at all. When seen in this light, the difficult adolescent becomes much easier to understand. And the goals of management become clear. These will be found in seeking methods whereby maladapting patients can regain their self-worth in better ways.

HIGH-RISK GROUPS

Identification of those who are most likely to respond to stress through maladaptive behavior is an issue of first importance. When staff members are alert to potential difficulty, they will not be taken off guard if it should occur and can meet the situation in more ordered terms. Awareness of just which youngsters may be at greatest risk allows for both the institution of preventive measures and the development of an advance management plan.

Preexisting Emotional Problems.   The adolescent who has a past history of coping poorly with stress often will respond to illness and hospitalization in much the same way. How any patient has previously dealt with anxiety is a reasonable indicator of what the staff may expect on the ward.

We again point to the importance of the psychosocial history, looking at the patient's functioning within his family, among peers, and at school. Does the youth have impulse control problems, frequently losing his or her temper? How is stress handled; is it effectively managed, or does the patient react in a disorganized way and become easily upset? How does the adolescent relate to agemates; is he isolated and a ''loner,'' or actively involved in peer group activities? What is the nature of his peer group; is it involved in delinquent behavior? Has there ever been a drug- or alcohol-abuse problem? Could the adolescent be considered seriously alienated from his family, in contrast to normal emancipation conflicts? To what degree can the patient confide in and communicate with parents? What are the causes of intrafamily arguments and how does the youth handle such events? How does he perform behaviorally and academically in a classroom setting, and what are his feelings about school and teachers (modified by those reality-based issues within the particular educational system itself)? What is the adolescent's dominant mood in relating to others: conforming or challenging, rebellious or compliant, leader or follower, shy and retiring or open and forward? The interviewer will certainly evolve her or his own questions and style. But the foregoing demonstrates the type of information needed and how to obtain it in relatively simple, direct, and concrete terms. Any adolescent who exhibits significant deviance from normal developmental expectancies in such matters should be considered at potential risk.

Adolescents with a past history of psychiatric treatment may also fall in this category. But great caution should be exercised in concluding that a patient will be a management problem on the basis of this piece of information alone. Not all such teen-agers are *de facto* disturbed. Even if they are, their problems may not necessarily interfere with adjusting to hospitalization. It is essential to know the reason for therapy before its significance for the youth's illness can be judged.

Agitated States.   Adolescents who arrive at the hospital in an agitated state comprise another group at risk. Here the patient's coping defenses are already seriously challenged and are in imminent danger of collapse. This type of response is most frequently seen in instances of unexpected injury or sudden illness where adjustment is profoundly compromised by the highly charged circumstances surrounding admission.

CASE 45.   A 17-year-old male was a passenger in an automobile accident that occurred late at night on a lonely road. He sustained a compound fracture of one leg but was otherwise unhurt, and he remained conscious throughout. His two companions, however, were instantly killed and the patient had been quite aware that they were at least gravely injured, if not dead. On arrival at the hospital he was highly agitated. Although he calmed down quite quickly in response to tranquilizing medication, convalescence was marked by a rather profound depression. Aware of this possibility in advance, the staff provided the boy with ample opportunity for ventilation of his feelings of helplessness, mourning for his lost companions, and dealing with his unrealistic fantasies of being somehow to blame. This was coupled with an activity program geared toward encouraging peer interaction. Although he was in traction, his bed was regularly transported to the adolescent day room. When seen a few months later he had made an excellent adjustment and was doing well.

Adolescents who come from families and subcultures where hysterical responses to stress are acceptable and even expected may also manifest agitation. Although such behavior can be most unnerving, it is usually quite adaptive and does not signify a behavior problem in the true sense of the word. In our experience adolescent girls of Hispanic background are particularly likely to act in this way.

Our greatest concern is reserved for agitated patients whose behavior is neither culturally determined nor justified by their medical condition. Here anxiety and distress derive from a much deeper cause. Adolescents appearing to fit this description warrant prompt evaluation for neurological or psychiatric disorders or for a toxic reaction to amphetamines, hallucinogens, or related drugs.

Injury and Guilt.   Trauma, a common cause of hospital admissions among adolescents, frequently occurs in the course of some rash, impulsive, or experimental deed. We consider all teen-agers admitted with this type of injury to be at risk, for profound guilt is inevitable when such a patient perceives that he is in some measure responsible for his own injured state. In turn, this often manifests itself in a "behavior problem" through depression, projection, or acting out.

Appropriate measures should always be taken to bring feelings of guilt out into the open where they can be dealt with in conscious and constructive terms. However, timing is important. In the acute phase of his condition the youth will generally have all that he can handle emotionally in contending with the biological threat itself; the issue of guilt may thus best be postponed until the youth is well into convalescence unless he initiates the discussion earlier himself.

Permanent Handicaps and Mutilations. The impact of irreversible injury or surgical and medical mutilation will be commented upon in some detail in chapters 10 and 11. We shall not dwell on the issue here. Suffice it to say that adolescents with permanent handicaps are particularly vulnerable and that maladaptive behavior occurs with some regularity during the hospital course of any patient who must revise his or her body image in seriously compromised terms.

CASE 46. A 19-year-old college student had taken an evening job in a liquor store to help pay his way through school. One night he was held up, and in resisting his assailant received the full blast of a shotgun straight in his face. Although he survived, his mouth and nose had been virtually destroyed. Many admissions for plastic surgery would be required. Understandably, his initial course was one of marked depression. While he was able to mingle freely with others as long as bandages hid his face, once these were removed he remained in his room isolated behind drawn bedside curtains. After several reconstructive procedures, although still rather grotesque, his mood changed. In an obvious effort to test out the acceptance of others and manipulatively gain their attention, he became incessantly voluble and gregarious.

In the beginning, staff and patients were most accepting and empathetic. But he made such a nuisance of himself and was so demanding of their time that tolerance gave way to impatience. He perceived this intolerance as stemming from his appearance rather than his behavior and once more went into retreat. These two patterns lurched back and forth until he was helped to understand the real reason he was being avoided. With time, he began to feel less diminished as a person, was able to adopt a more moderate schedule of socialization, and was once again welcomed by his peers.

But the period between his many admissions was infinitely more painful and he was always devastated by an impending discharge. While the youth could deal with his appearance in the protective and accepting environment of the hospital, this was not possible in the less tolerant outside world. As the time to leave approached, he developed a host of assorted physical symptoms and took to his bed. While at home he remained inside his house, cut off from all congress with past friends. It would undoubtedly be some time before these reality-based depressive reactions would give way to a more compensatory defense. And the degree to which he will be able to accomplish this may finally depend on the success of surgery itself.

COMMON BEHAVIORAL THEMES

A maladapting patient may choose from a variety of behavioral alternatives. We shall look not so much at their outward manifestations as at what they represent. While one can provide temporary, palliative relief for the symptoms themselves, these will persist until their genesis is discovered. While aggressive attacks, treatment refusals, sexual provocations, or running away can each be temporarily contained, the underlying anxiety will continue to provoke problems until the cause can be identified and relieved.

Inner-Directed Behaviors.   A patient may emotionally retreat when he feels he can no longer contend with the outside world. This may be either because of the magnitude of the threat, real or fantasied, or because he has not sufficient inner resources available to meet even a modest amount of stress in any other way. The adolescent thus erects a protective shield through which no outside insults can penetrate. Inner-directed behavior also often represents the internalization of aggressive feelings directed at another that cannot be acted upon without intolerable guilt. But whatever their derivation, these behaviors tend to restrict the patient's ability to relate to others significantly, depriving him of the associated boost to his self-esteem. Moreover, it can be much more difficult to move into positive, compensatory coping from a withdrawn position than when one starts from an outer-directed mode. These behaviors are often accompanied by regression, and the quiet, retreating youth may be infantile and demanding as well.

Depression and withdrawal. Nearly every adolescent patient normally experiences some degree of depression and withdrawal during the course of his or her hospitalization. For the most part, however, this is transient and situationally related, serving a valid function in conserving emotional energy at times of high biological stress. But a "problem" exists when this mood persists beyond a reasonable length of time or is inappropriate to the circumstances at hand.

CASE 47. A 15-year-old girl was admitted for the surgical removal of an enlarging and ugly mole on her cheek. In her own mind's eye she had come to see this blemish as the cause of all her troubles in relating to peers. And she was indeed having considerable difficulty in dating, tending to be shy and withdrawn. She arrived at the hospital eagerly anticipating the results of the procedure and was most cooperative preoperatively. But a normal degree of postsurgical regression failed to resolve and she remained quite depressed. It ultimately emerged that she had unconsciously magnified the distortion in her appearance in order to ward off long-standing anxieties about members of the opposite sex. As long as she could perceive herself as ugly, she felt safe. But, when this solution was no longer viable following surgery, becoming regressed and withdrawn was the best she could do.

Organically impaired mental functions. Patients who have suffered from central nervous system injury or disease, are under the effects of drugs, or are toxic from some other cause may also exhibit withdrawn behavior. In each instance this is biologically mediated, and management primarily rests in identifying and treating the underlying cause. Careful mental status examinations, often serially done, are most important here. A major challenge rests in differentiating organic from psychogenic depression when the causal agent is obscure. Such diagnostic confusions are particularly apt to occur in instances of covert drug abuse or unrecognized head trauma.

Borderline psychosis. Clearly psychotic adolescents are discussed in the next chapter, but we mention them here in completing our differential diagnosis of inner-directed behaviors, for a borderline psychosis is not always readily recognizable. Although uncommon, the possibility of psychosis should be considered in patients who seem remote and who have difficulty in establishing affective relationships. One senses a certain strangeness and distance, and staff members tend to experience considerable difficulty in "tuning in" to the youth's "wave length" and in mobilizing empathy. Under the stress of illness and hospitalization, these qualities may become yet more pronounced or even herald a frank psychotic break.

Outer-Directed Behaviors.   This category includes defensive behaviors that are targeted at others and that deal with anxiety through action rather than self-insultation. These types of problem are particularly disruptive, frequently precipitating crises on the ward. Outer-directed behaviors not only are difficult to manage but also tend to entrap staff and other patients, provoking them to anger or avoidance.

CASE 48.   A 17-year-old boy had been born with ambiguous genitalia. At one month of age he was identified as male and so reared. Surgery corrected hypospadias and a scrotal anomaly, but his microphallus remained. Puberty was entirely normal with full masculinization and normal testicular size. But the penis measured little more than five centimeters in length even in the erect state. He was now admitted for further attempts to correct this deficiency.

Although the boy dated and was active in sports, he carefully avoided revealing his anatomical abnormality to anyone else. And, although he masturbated regularly and did have an ejaculate, he had never attempted sexual intercourse.

But it was obvious that he vigorously overcompensated for his feelings of sexual inadequacy. For he was exceedingly provocative. He usually went about the ward without a pajama top, and subtly flexed his muscles at every chance. He assumed a proprietary manner over both student and younger staff nurses and wished them to heed his every beck and call. On several occasions he went so far as to proposition several of the nurses and a female patient, telling them how good he was in bed. He managed to thoroughly embarrass and discomfort both patients and staff, who responded (quite naturally) by vigorous avoidance.

In managing this problem, not only did the ward team have to set limits on the boy's behavior and help him to cope better, but they also had to contend with this clear threat to their own professional equanimity and self-control.

Similar outer-directed behavior patterns may have different derivations. A patient's abusive belligerence can variably stem from impulse control difficulties, manipulation attempts, or the edge of panic. Moreover, a given behavior pattern may be multidetermined, and an adolescent who refuses his or her medication could be responding from both depression and acting out. Management will have some variations on basic themes depending upon the underlying cause.

Impulse disorders. Some adolescents seem never to have learned to contain or control their instinctive aggressive drives. Such patients have a singularly low frustration tolerance and are quick to anger when they feel exploited, neglected, or unfairly treated. Often uncertain of their own self-worth, these youngsters experience an exaggerated need to defend the ''territorialism'' of their inner selves. An impulse disorder inevitably will have been manifested in the past. School performance may be particularly telling, with abundant reports of poor temper control and aggressive outbursts in response to minimal provocations. The patient himself will also often speak of how easily he becomes angry and simply has to lash out.

Impulse disorders should not be confused with outbursts in the face of circumstances that would try any man's soul, and some differentiation must be made between true maladaptation and a valid situational response. An adolescent who loses his temper after repeated postponement of anticipated surgery, endless waits on an uncomfortable stretcher in the radiology suite, or a clattering of bedpans at seven in the morning after a fitful and restless night's sleep is entitled to express his impatience. To be passively accepting and not exhibit anger under such conditions would be unusual indeed.

While the commonest manifestation of poor impulse control is an outburst of temper, elopement is another alternative. Impulsive adolescents whose internalized guilt is sufficient to block an aggressive response may have no option but running away. In either case, the motivation is an inability to tolerate stress to any significant degree or to interact with it in more effective terms.

Provocative and manipulative behaviors. These behaviors are manifested not only in aggression and elopement but also in a wide variety of other attention-seeking devices; monopolization of staff time, repetitive and exaggerated complaints and demands, noncompliance with and sabotage of treatment, and sexually seductive behavior are but a few. In contrast to impulse disorders, the underlying motivation here is not frustration intolerance but the patient's need to seek reassurance of his continued worth and to know that he will not be irrevocably devalued or abandoned.

CASE 49.   A 13-year-old boy suffered a cerebral hemorrhage as a newborn infant and required a ventriculopleural shunt. He had done remarkably well over the ensuing years, and up to the time of the present admission had had no further difficulty. Indeed, the family had all but forgotten about this problem.

About two weeks before admission, the boy began to experience severe headaches, double vision, and vomiting. A neurological evaluation confirmed the initial impression that increased intracranial pressure had returned. Surgery found the membrane surrounding his old hemorrhage still intact and fluid had started collecting again. The offending tissue was removed, and the shunt revised. There was little likelihood that his problem would recur.

During convalescence the boy was all over the ward monopolizing anyone he could and talked incessantly about all sorts of trivia. When rebuffed in these endeavors, he increased his efforts even more. Indeed, he came to be viewed as a real pest and nuisance by all, stretching the patience of the ward staff almost beyond endurance.

A problem-solving conference was held and, in evaluating the situation, what seemed to be the prime problem came to light. The boy's parents were also having great difficulty in handling the recurrence of their son's disease. This was manifest in diffuse anxiety, disorganization and overprotectiveness. In turn, the patient became convinced that his parents' shifting attitudes portended a grave prognosis for himself. In monopolizing the attention of others, he was seeking to manipulate them in an effort to demonstrate that he at least was in control, even if his parents were not, and to resecure a relationship of being seen as "okay."

Therapeutic goals were primarily aimed at helping his parents to see how their own exaggerated distress was affecting their son and at regaining a sense of proportion. As this occurred, they were enabled to relate to him as they had in the past. In addition, the medical situation and its good prognosis were carefully reviewed with the boy himself. Well-defined limits were set on his behavior in firm but kindly terms; and he was helped to look at his own basic fears through talking with the ward social worker and participating in regular ward discussion groups.

Attention-seeking behavior is common in adolescence, when narcissistic and individuating drives are characteristically expressed in somewhat provocative terms. But some teen-agers' behavior is far in excess of this normal and expected range and poses a true problem. These youngsters, frequently subjects of early childhood deprivation, have little basis for trust and relate to others in a manipulative manner for much of their lives. Attentions from parents or other family members may have been forthcoming only through deliberate provocations. While a quiet and compliant child can easily be ignored, it is difficult not to pay attention to the one who somehow engenders anger or learns to exploit parental guilt feelings. And even if such maneuvers prompt contact only in abusive or punitive terms, this is still far preferable to no contact at all.

CASE 50. A 15-year-old female was admitted for the first of a two-stage procedure to repair bilateral congenital strabismus. This had been quite ignored by her family over the years, until their hand was forced in this matter subsequent to a teacher's report of poor vision. The girl had a long history of rejection and abuse, and had indeed been an unwanted child. Her alcoholic mother had handed her over to the care of an aunt who wanted her even less. Shunted off into the corner, the girl quickly learned that the only way she could gain any attention at all was through creating a fuss, even though this produced both verbal and physical abuse.

While on the ward she was most taken aback by the kindness and consideration of the staff. She found this almost overwhelming and impossible to accept. Not only was it difficult for her to trust caring and warmth, but she also felt intolerably guilty at not having a valid target for her deep and abiding anger at having been so deprived. In consequence, she rather deliberately set out to make herself obnoxious as possible in order to engender the kind of hostile reaction that she found so familiar and with which she was comfortable.

Fortunately, there was a spark of awareness and desire for something better, and the girl was finally able to establish a positive relationship with the ward recreational worker that continued long after discharge through the technique of enlisting her as a volunteer. (She was in fact most able in working with younger children.) Initially, this was a highly testing situation in which the girl was both belligerent and demanding. Then it moved into a self-deprecatory phase in which she constantly voiced her own sense of worthlessness and attempted to gain the worker's concurrence. Gradually a trust relationship did develop, with the girl much more able to be open and straightforward with others as well. Some months later admission for repair of the second eye was well tolerated and uneventful.

Acting out. The manifestations of acting out are virtually identical with those cited before. In many respects this device is closely related to provocative behavior, and often both coexist. But in this instance the underlying motivation is not quite so much the engendering of some sort of responsiveness and attention from others as it is a quite simple and direct assertion of self and statement of protest. If falls somewhere between the urgent lashing out and self-protective measures of an impulse disorder and the specific attention-seeking goals of manipulation. Its intent is primarily to reclaim command, to resecure a sense of self and individuation, and to protect from inner feelings of an impending defensive collapse. How others will react to such behavior is of less importance to the patient than how it helps him resecure a sense of self-esteem on his own.

As with provocative and manipulative modes, acting out may be largely situationally related. This would be the case for a teen-ager who is defiant and angry in response to enforced dependency, curtailed drives toward mastery and control, or the threat of possible permanent disability. On the other hand, this may also represent a primary defense deriving from early life experiences as a protest against all the injustice and unfairness to which the adolescent feels victim. The ward staff will need to sort out carefully what is truly maladaptive and inconsistent with good care and what is transient and tolerable.

CASE 51.   A 17-year-old high school football star was admitted for the surgical correction of a persistent back injury. Preoperatively, he seemed confident and self-assured. But following his operation he continued to be regressive and demanding far longer than normally encountered. The nursing staff felt particularly stressed by his unremitting requests for analgesia and continuous calls for nothing much at all.

It was decided that his day nurse would sit down and talk with him at some length, pointing out the problem and asking him why he seemed so upset. The answers were loud and clear. First, the youth had been quite unprepared for the level of pain and discomfort that he would experience. This had been far beyond what he had learned to tolerate in the usual exigencies of his chosen sport and had been most frightening. Second, he heartily resented having to be in bed and immobilized. Third, he was not entirely sure what his future held and whether he would still be able to play on the team. And, last, his girlfriend had neither visited nor called and there had been no answer when he telephoned her home. Collectively, these matters had become an insuperable barrier to his coping more effectively, although he could have undoubtedly handled one or two alone.

In meeting this problem, his doctor carefully reviewed his course and prognosis proffering every reasonable expectation that he would play football again, though perhaps not for a while. Ventilation was encouraged by his regular nurse within a climate of empathetic acceptance of his discomfort and frustration. His bed was frequently moved to the day room for social congress. And the social worker managed to discover that his girlfriend had unexpectedly been called out of town because of a relative's death. Within several days his outlook significantly improved.

Panic. This pattern of behavior is primarily manifest in fight-fright-flight reactions, and encompasses such matters as combative outbursts, diffuse hysteria, and precipitous elopements. All basically reflect the fact that the patient has become overwhelmed by anxiety and can no longer cope with it in other than these highly primitive terms. This is not a customary or long-standing behavior, as the former alternatives may be but, rather, is a highly limited and circumscribed response to unusually threatening circumstances. A precipitating and causal event always antecedes panic. This may vary anywhere from suddenly hearing distressing news or the imposition of unprepared-for surgery to the performance of a particularly long and painful procedure. In other instances the source of panic may not be external, but within the patient himself and his distorted fantasies or mistaken beliefs about something that outwardly seems quite benign.

Anyone may become victim to panic, given the right set of circumstances. Undoubtedly, each of us would run as fast as he could if he was charged by a large, roaring lion and had no gun. In many respects, when and if a patient panics depends on just how big he sees his own particular "lion" to be, and whether he is armed or not. Prevention lies in this latter point. For adolescents who are well equipped with knowledge about what is happening and why will be much more prepared to handle threatening situations effectively than those who are taken off guard.

GENERAL MANAGEMENT PRINCIPLES

Our basic management approach for adolescent patients in general also has both preventive and therapeutic benefits for those who are behaviorally disturbed. In many instances one need do little more. For frequently such difficulties arise from the stress of illness and injury compounded by an inappropriate hospital milieu or staff response. When either of these factors is eliminated, the patient is often able to cope with the other reasonably well. But we also recommend that additional measures be taken with teen-agers who are in high risk or who seem already to be having more problems than most.

A well-defined and coordinated plan is essential. Clear objectives need to be established as to precise staff roles and how they will be integrated. When the separate skills of nursing, social work, recreational therapy, education, liaison psychiatry, and medicine are joined, no one professional ends up having to carry the burden of a difficult teen-ager all alone. A circle of care supports the patient on all sides, and possibilities for individual staff members reacting in unconstructive ways are minimized.

CASE 52.   A 15-year-old male with ulcerative colitis had been refusing to comply with therapeutic recommendations. At home there was an unending series of intrafamily rows over this matter, and his parents were in frantic despair over their inability to control their son's behavior. At school he was either belligerent or truant and his teachers considered him little more than a trouble maker. They found it difficult to believe that his many requests to go to the bathroom or his frequent absences were all in fact medically mediated. And in some measure they were quite right. Further, he had terminated psychotherapy and refused to go any more.

His primary physician was attempting to handle this situation alone, but was both short on time and uncomfortable in dealing with the boy's emotional problems without psychiatric assistance. The doctor managed matters in somewhat coercive and authoritarian terms, telling the patient that he would have to have his colon removed and a colostomy if he did not comply. The doctor empathized far more with the parents' frustration than with the boy and his need for denial and acting out. In consequence, the patient felt that no one was on his side and became even more angry, rebellious, and resistant to therapy until he became too ill to protest any more.

In the ward team conference the following plan was evolved. The adolescent medicine specialist joined the primary physician in direct patient management with the aim of establishing a transference relationship and being exclusively on the patient's side. The social worker assumed this same type of supportive role with the parents. In consequence, the primary physician was no longer put in the ambiguous position of having to meet the emotional needs of both sides at once. The recreational therapist involved the boy in constructive group activity, encouraged ventilation, and served as his advocate while on the ward. It was much easier and less threatening for the youth to express his anger and resentment to someone who was not directly involved in his medical care. The ward teacher met with his school and relayed the doctors' directions on what his health problem required in the way of bathroom privileges and possible absences, relieving a good bit of hostility on this front. In addition, she helped set up a less taxing schedule with extra time for him to receive help in school with his lagging homework and missed assignments. And, while definite limits were set as to what was and was not acceptable behavior on the ward, nursing still provided a great deal of room for the patient's own self-determination and control within these boundaries. In a relatively short period of time, the patient's anger and rebelliousness abated a bit, the parents became less coercive, and a better level of control of the disease was achieved.

A number of helpful devices can be employed within the general framework of the team approach. In essence these are variations on basic management themes, modified to meet the needs of troubled adolescents. With proper selection and application, according to the nature of the behavior at hand, these techniques can contribute substantially to the effective management of a difficult youth.

Ventilation.   Simply helping the patient talk about what is upsetting him and "getting it off his chest" is therapeutic in and of itself. The continual repression of anger, fear, or sadness requires the diversion of emotional energy away from the proper business of coping with these feelings in more direct and constructive terms. Ventilation can be accomplished through either individual or group sessions. In the former instance, the therapist need not be a mental health specialist; any ward team member can serve—nurses, recreation personnel, social workers, physicians, or even the ward teacher. Each in turn may be the one a troubled adolescent feels he or she can confide in and talk to best.

Although the youth should feel free to express his concerns to any or all staff members according to his needs and desires, the primary responsibility for encouraging and promoting ventilation should be vested in a single professional. The choice of just who should fill this spot depends on a number of factors: who has the most frequent contact with the patient, who feels the most comfortable with the problem, who relates to the adolescent best, and, in a most pragmatic vein, who in fact can manage to squeeze in the time.

Sitting down with the patient in a quiet place and proferring the observation that he or she seems to be having a good bit of difficulty in coping with his or her condition often serves as a good opening. Nonspecific inquiries such as "How are things going?" or "Do you have anything on your mind?" should be avoided. These tend to have the *pro forma* quality of the traditional telephone greeting of "Hello, how are you?" to which the expected reply is "Fine, thank you," whether things are fine or not. Adolescents who have problems in relating to others are particularly apt to be quite unsure of whether such concerns are honestly meant. Teen-agers can also have considerable difficulty in expressing feelings and may need some assistance in formulating their concerns. Far better introduce the topic in quite specific terms: "You seem very angry [depressed, upset]. I'd like to hear about what you think is causing this, so together we can find a way for you to feel better." An observation about the behavior pattern itself can also be useful: "I think you must be very worried about something, or else I know you wouldn't be making things so difficult by being so aggressive [hostile, demanding]."

Not all young people are sufficiently trusting to reveal their feelings in the intimacy of a one-to-one situation, regardless of the skill of the professional involved. Group "rap" sessions can be highly effective for these patients. And the economy offered to a busy staff by working with several youngsters at once is an added bonus. Group settings offer the patient the example, support, and encouragement of other adolescents who have already become adept at expressing their thoughts and concerns. And often these will be reassuringly similar to the patient's own. Moreover, group therapy among teen-agers firmly ties in with the developmental importance of the peer group. We shall not define group dynamics here, but we do recommend that these sessions be led by staff persons experienced in such techniques. The social worker, adolescent medicine specialist, recreational therapist, and liaison psychologist or psychiatrist will usually be the ones most often involved.

Allaying Cognitive Distortion.   We have often spoken of how easy it is for adolescent patients to misinterpret what they hear, see, or sense. Once again, we make a firm plea for appropriate and well-timed explanations of what is happening and why, what is planned for the immediate and long-range future, and what outcome is anticipated.

CASE 53.   A 14-year-old male with osteomyelitis of one knee shared a room with a youth newly diagnosed as having advanced Hodgkin's disease. While the first boy was doing well and expected to recover fully, his roommate's case was considerably more dire, and on daily rounds the former was given quite short shrift, being no longer cause for much concern. The lengthy, guarded, and whispered discussions around the door all pertained to the other. But the youth with osteomyelitis had not been told of his excellent progress in clear and well-defined terms, and he came to believe that all the grave considerations he overheard were about himself. Muttered statements about impending surgery were interpreted as portending the possible loss of his leg. This distortion was further supported by the evidence of his continuing intravenous therapy. While this was a routine measure in the treatment of his disease, the boy saw this only as an indicator that things were not going well at all.

He became increasingly agitated, hostile, and uncooperative. On one occasion following rounds (and a particularly long and worried conversation about the roommate), the boy became frankly panicked, pulled out his IV, and took off down the hall with all the ward staff in hot pursuit. He was told that if he did not behave himself he would surely become sick and might even lose his leg. It was an attempt to shock him into compliance, but of course they only fed into his basic fears and simply made matters worse.

We shall not belabor the issue here. Suffice it to say that adolescent patients need to know much more about their care and prognosis than they are usually told. Explanations of these matters are often too technical, too infrequent, and too brief. The failure to recognize this point may not only promote maladaptive behavior all on its own, but will certainly compound matters for those who are primarily distressed on some other count.

Staff-Patient Relationship.   Troubled adolescents often have difficulty in relating to the staff through the ordinary processes of "routine" care, tending to see them in controlling and punitive terms. We thus consider it essential that at least one member of the ward team develop a strong relationship with an emotionally distressed youth, with the goals of becoming the patient's advocate, encouraging a transference relationship, fostering identification, and serving as a role model.

If the problem patient is to come to a helpful understanding of what is happening to him, or be able to look at and resolve his basic fears and gain insight into how his behavior interferes with his getting well or the rights of others, some sort of a trust relationship must come about first. This is often best accomplished through the designated staff member's first taking a firm and empathetic advocacy role in representing the youth's concerns and unmet needs to others. In this initial stage there is no attempt to modify the behavior itself but, rather, to convince the patient that at least one person is on his side. This approach usually allows matters to move easily into ventilation and finally into a more definitive and therapeutic exploration of the behavioral problem itself. These steps can often be carried out by a single staff member. But sometimes a psychiatric consultation is indicated. The patient should always be truthfully told of this need, and that a psychiatrist will be coming to talk with him soon.

Limit Setting. Up to this point, some may feel that our methods of managing maladapting youths are excessively permissive and wholly overlook discipline. But such an assumption is in error. We do not condone an adolescent's unrestricted carrying on in any way that *significantly* interferes with his own care or that of others. Firm limits on truly detrimental behavior must be set.

Just how to exert control over an unruly, headstrong, and rebellious youth can be perplexing. What sanctions can one impose upon an adolescent that will indeed result in compliant behavior? The answer is none; and nothing can be more futile than attempting to modify a teen-ager's behavior through punitive and coercive means. Short of being chained to the bedstead or locked up in his room forever, he can manage to outflank virtually every move if he so chooses. In consequence, ward staff members are apt to resort to either of two extremes. At one end is attempting to force the youth's compliance by some sort of restrictive and coercive emotional "chains," and at the other is the tendency to avoid the matter entirely, not wishing to test out just who is really "in charge" for fear they will lose.

Yet a disruptive adolescent must be advised of what he is doing and of its unacceptability. But the affective mood surrounding this communication is critical; these matters must be conveyed in concerned and honest terms by one who is neither judgmental and autocratic on the one hand nor intimidated by the patient on the other. Limit setting consists of a calm but firm announcement that the patient simply will not be allowed to continue to disrupt the ward or to harm himself or others, that the staff is sure he would like to do better, and that everyone is there to help.

In many instances the adolescent will recognize that he is his own worst enemy and may even go so far as to welcome these external controls when proffered in an empathetic way. But it is also true that these limits will inevitably require continual reinforcement. The staff can expect to have to repeat the message many times, and should not lose patience prematurely.

Minor tranquilizers or the phenothiazides sometimes can be helpful adjuncts by diminishing the patient's underlying anxiety to the point where he feels less pressured to misbehave. But we are firmly opposed to the use of such medication when the primary purpose is simply to contain the patient in a pharmacological straitjacket for the convenience of the staff. Except as an urgently needed protective measure, tranquilizers should be employed only as a carefully considered component of a well-thought-out overall plan. Just which drug should be used depends on both the severity of the distress and the familiarity of the ward staff with the various agents themselves. There is a veritable army of psychotropic medications and the physician should use the ones that he or she knows best. We ourselves generally prefer diazepam (Valium) and chlorpromazine (Thorazine).

In some extreme instances, a behavior problem will pose a serious and imminent danger to the youth himself, to essential medical care, or to the safety of others. When alternative methods fail in these circumstances, outright bodily containment may be necessary. While we consider the use of physical force with a patient to be abhorrent, this course has to be seen as infinitely preferable to allowing serious harm to be done. This need is most apt to arise in instances of panic, loss of impulse control, suicidal attempts, or frank psychotic breaks.

Limit setting can be truly effective only in combination with at least some of the other facets of an overall management approach. Otherwise this step only adds more fuel to the fire of the adolescent's discontent. Moreover, this measure can only work when the adolescent perceives that it is validly and fairly imposed.

Environmental Involvement.   Peer socialization, activity programs, and resumption of schooling all afford opportunities for deterring or alleviating maladaptive behavior. An adolescent's normal need for peer group acceptance, mastery and control, and enhancement of self-esteem is even more heightened in those who are least able to cope. Patients with outer-directed behavior disturbances find particular benefits here. For impulsive, provocative, or acting-out youths tend to find it difficult to express themselves in verbal terms.

One should not overlook the benefits of role reversal, wherein the youth, in part, becomes a caretaker rather than care recipient by being given responsibility for helping with younger children or assigned some other helpful task on the ward. We have found this to be particularly useful for adolescents who are self-destructive and manipulative.

CASE 54. A 16-year-old male with asthma was readmitted in status asthmaticus for the fifth time in a year. Although he had a full array of medications at home and was supposed to be receiving desensitization shots, he constantly managed to "forget" these things. The boy lived with an aunt, as his parents were deceased, but neither she nor any other relative really wanted him, and he knew this. The only place he felt secure and accepted was in the hospital, and in failing to take his medication he was able to remain here a good bit of the time.

During this latest stay, special efforts were geared toward helping the patient establish a good relationship with the ward recreational therapist and to accept the psychotherapeutic interventions of the fellow in adolescent medicine. When up and about, he was encouraged to help out with the younger children, as it had been noted that he was excellent with them on his own initiative. After discharge, he was invited to become a regular hospital volunteer several afternoons a week, still under the aegis of the recreational therapist, but now in an employer-employee relationship. He thoroughly enjoyed his work and was responsible and reliable throughout. In this way he was able to maintain his contact with those he cared for most—the hospital staff—but now in constructive rather than destructive terms. He regularly followed his medical regimen and for the first time in months became symptom free.

Specific Measures in Depression. Depressed and withdrawn adolescents may need particular help to reengage with their environment. In essence, this consists of drawing the patient out of his isolation and retreat by offering frequent opportunities for contact. Depending on the depth of the mood, therapy may consist only of reassuring statements, holding a hand, or sitting quietly at the bedside for a while with a youngster who mutely turns his head away; or it may include the empathetic verbal sharing of feelings of despair with an adolescent who is willing to talk.

In other instances these measures may be more action oriented in finding ways to help the adolescent leave the isolation of his room and reengage with his peers; or become involved in some activity that provides an opportunity for him to work through his feelings and invoke compensation. At times this may manifest itself in unexpected terms.

CASE 55.   A 14-year-old gang member had been stabbed several times in the abdomen during a street fight. He had sustained penetrating wounds through the stomach, liver, and pancreas. Emergency surgery closed these defects, but his postoperative course was complicated by both a chemical and bacterial peritonitis. It was several weeks before he was sufficiantly well to be up and about. From the outset the boy was withdrawn and isolated. Initially, this was thought to be an appropriate consequence of his biological condition and the valid need to conserve energy. But, as convalescence progressed, the boy made little effort to resume normal activity and remained markedly depressed.

Further investigation revealed that he had been living with his elderly grandparents who had recently come to find his emancipation strivings more than they could contend with. In attempting to control his behavior, they had become increasingly restrictive and punitive. In response, the boy had run away and sought refuge at the home of a friend who had then involved him in the neighborhood gang. His feelings of anger and alienation about his grandparents, the belief that his injury was somehow a retribution for his running away, and the valid perceptions of just how ill he was all contributed to his depression.

Ultimately, he was coaxed out of his bed and into the adolescent day room for peer activity. But he slipped away, only to be later found in the younger children's playroom down the hall. Here he was carrying out a "successful" surgical procedure in the doll corner set aside for this purpose. And for a number of days he could always be found here. But it was not long before he had apparently worked through his regression and returned to be with his peers and participate in more age-appropriate activity.

Initial efforts at involving depressed and retreating adolescents may well seem ineffective. At times they may even be rejected in a hostile outburst. But if such responses are seen as simply the best that the adolescent can do to defend himself at the moment, staff need not succumb to feelings of frustration or even anger at being rebuffed. Continued gentle efforts along these lines will usually be productive, given enough time.

Specific Measures in Panic. Evidence of increasingly agitated behavior should alert the staff to the potential of impending panic. This is often a premonitory sign of the fact that the patient is being stressed to the utmost and has few residual inner reserves. In instances of both incipient and outright panic, the most important first step is to identify and remove the precipitating cause, or at least set it temporarily aside. This will then give the patient a chance to gather his or her defenses together in better form. When these measures are ineffective or the causal event obscure, the prompt administration of a tranquilizer may be indicated. Rational appeals or discussions are pointless at this time, for they will not be heeded at all. And, for the same reason, any ventilation or exploration of the problem should be postponed until the patient has regained his composure to some degree.

It is also helpful to recognize that the adolescent will be just as disconcerted by his own defensive collapse and failure to cope in more organized terms as he was by the precipitating threat itself. Basic drives are all in the direction of establishing some sort of emotional equilibrium, and panic almost always has an inherently self-limiting quality.

CASE 56.   A seemingly well-adjusted 13-year-old boy was admitted for investigation of a persistent fever. Diagnostic efforts required frequent blood tests. As each was about to be drawn, he became increasingly agitated and pleaded for its postponement. On the morning of the third day the house officer approached with a larger than customary syringe. The boy panicked and smashed it out of his hand, kicked an assisting nurse in the stomach, ran to the bathroom, and locked himself in.

The nurse quietly went to the door, the rest of the staff having been enjoined to stay out. She called to the boy, reassuring him that blood would not be drawn that day, and asked that he come out. She also told him how the staff understood and sympathized with his distress and that they were not angry, nor would he be punished. After about fifteen minutes the boy calmed down sufficiently to unlock the door and allowed the nurse to take him back to bed and settle him down. (In the interim all possibly threatening equipment had been removed from his room.) The doctor briefly put his head in the door with a pleasant greeting and further assurances that everything was "okay." A little later on, when the youth was calmed down, the social worker began to talk about what had happened. It was discovered that the patient believed his strength and power rested in his blood and that as this was gradually being drawn out he would become weaker and weaker and perhaps even die. These thoughts related to an earlier time of childhood iron-deficiency anemia and his mother's persistent overprotective attitude. Even when cured, she constantly importuned the boy to eat well to "keep his blood up and stay strong." Further, she had always seen to it that he took Geritol, and the boy was most familiar with its advertisements of curing "tired" blood.

These thoughts were countered by a careful explanation in correction of his misinformation, by taking him to the hematology lab and letting him see blood smear slides and the actual performance of chemical tests, and by encouraging him to talk with other patients who had had a similar amount of blood drawn without consequent harm.

While his behavior undoubtedly stemmed from an even deeper fear than the simplified explanation offered above, these measures were quite sufficient to enable him to be most cooperative throughout his stay. No cause for his fever was uncovered, and it ultimately disappeared all on its own. After discharge, he returned to his former well-adjusted state and it was not deemed necessary to intervene with any further psychiatric investigations at this time.

Psychiatric Liaison and Consultation.   We fully realize the difficulties encountered by busy or inexperienced staff in mounting all the preceding interventive steps. We strongly recommend that the services of the liaison psychiatrist or psychologist be regularly employed in planning the management approach for any behaviorally disturbed adolescent. Nor will all the problems posed by maladapting teen-agers be axiomatically resolved by these methods. Youths with long-standing histories of trouble are particularly resistant to even the best of efforts. And when these measures fail, as inevitably they sometimes will, definitive psychiatric evaluation and intervention will be required.

SEXUALLY PROVOCATIVE BEHAVIORS

Up to this point we have not addressed the specific ways in which behavioral disturbances may be expressed, and have already stated that we consider this less important than the underlying intent. But sexually provocative behavior is an exception because of the distress that this topic invariably engenders among professional and administrative staff alike. Possibilities for sexual acting out are inevitably cited as a major deterring factor among those thinking of establishing a mixed adolescent ward.

The vast majority of adolescents are quite well aware of the appropriate settings for the expression of physical affection, and the hospital is seldom seen as a valid place to "make out." While teen-agers are impulsive and experimental at times, one must also credit them with at least some measure of good judgment and common sense. Moreover, most ill or injured young people are far too preoccupied with themselves and their health to be concerned with sexual conquests—nor do they wish to reveal humiliating bodily deficiencies to others.

Additional restraints rest in the fact that many of the medical processes attendant to hospitalization are also erotically charged, prompting particularly strong defenses against this seduction. One need only consider the highly intimate bodily invasions that occur during physical examinations, nursing care, and the like to establish this point. In consequence, adolescents tend to be considerably more restrained in their sexual behavior than usual, protecting themselves from losing control of their own aroused feelings. We firmly support the concept of the mixed adolescent ward and offer reassurance to those embarking on this step that heavy petting or outright sexual intercourse among hospitalized teen-agers is a remarkably rare event.

But it would be a significant mistake to deny the fact that adolescents are indeed highly invested in and preoccupied with their developing sexual identity. These concerns are even more enhanced when a major illness or injury supervenes. Teen-agers in the hospital will most certainly make every effort to resecure their sense of masculinity or femininity during convalescence through exploring whether they can still attract members of the opposite sex. In this context, boys and girls generally enjoy socializing together on the ward just as much as they do on the outside. (Indeed, failing to reactivate these interests while getting well is developmentally inappropriate, and should in and of itself suggest that there may be something wrong.) But this does not mean that patients will inevitably act on these drives and spend their convalescence leaping from bed to bed.

Masturbatory activity may be encountered from time to time. But this almost always occurs when the patient's privacy is unexpectedly invaded (and a knock on a convalescent's closed door is always a wise precaution). Masturbation is a normal event in the life of the adolescent and, when privately carried out, is not inconsistent with hospitalization where it serves as a reassuring exploration of biological and sexual intactness. We consider this issue to be primarily a problem for staff sensibilities, not for the patient himself.

Still, sexual encounters among patients on the ward do occur occasionally. But in our experience there are usually clear premonitory signs that should sound the alert. Teen-aged girls (out of cultural determinants of feminine attractiveness) are most often the ones to set the stage through rather clear and overt seductions. Those who wear sheer and low-cut nightgowns, inadequately robe themselves, go about with buttons open and ties undone, or lie in bed in a revealing pose warrant close observation. Firm but kindly limits on what is worn outside the room and a direct discussion about the inappropriateness of such behavior on a hospital ward are indicated. In addition, other more acceptable methods of gaining attention and resecuring sexual identity should be invoked. But sometimes this behavior is habitual and so resistant to change that staff can do little more than keep out a wary and careful eye.

Occasionally, one encounters a patient who has been having sexual intercourse with his or her dating partner on the outside, and the couple may wish to resume this behavior during visiting hours. We do not either condemn or condone premarital coitus *per se*. But such behavior is inappropriate in the confines of the general hospital ward because of the lack of privacy. This prohibition rests more in avoiding offending the staff, other patients, or visitors than because of this necessarily being harmful for the young couple themselves. This latter point is a matter for individualized assessment based on matters quite extraneous to the circumstances of hospitalization itself. However, this is quite another matter for patients in long-term chronic disease or rehabilitation facilities. We need to give hard thought about providing opportunities for mature and loving young couples to have sexual intercourse when they face institutionalization for many months or years.

CONCLUSION

In this chapter we have examined behavior patterns that frequently cause difficulties on the adolescent ward, identified patients at greatest risk, and suggested some helpful preventive and therapeutic measures. But we must insert a final note of caution about seeing any given patient in such simplified and dissected terms. In most instances the manifestations of behavioral difficulties are multidetermined.

Further, while reactions primarily precipitated by events surrounding illness and hospitalization are usually quite amenable to our management approach, long-standing maladaptations stemming from early life may be much more resistant. At times the staff will need to accept the fact that they can do little about a difficult teen-ager except to contain his behavior as best they can and try to engage him in some form of long-range psychotherapy. On rarer occasions one must also accept the fact that not even this can be accomplished, and a speedy discharge may be the only resort.

To avoid ending on such a pessimistic note, let us add that most adolescents, even at their most impossible, will in some measure respond to tolerance, empathy, and reasonable limit setting. And, in making this possible, it is the staff's responsibility to recognize the futility of either overidentification or an adversarial approach, and to engage the adolescent in a collaborative venture in getting him well. Sharing the burden of the difficult youth through a well-conceived and disciplined team approach will go far toward helping each professional achieve this goal.

chapter ten

**Particularly Difficult Situations
and Stressful Procedures**

Some special situations inevitably pose singular stresses to an adolescent's psychological and biological integrity and place greater burdens on the staff. Awareness of the issues involved and specific attention to them in management will be helpful in effectively meeting the heightened needs of all concerned.

SENSORY DEPRIVATIONS

The recovery room, intensive care unit, and medical isolation all offer significant potential for emotional decompensation consequent to the effects of metabolic disturbance and sensory deprivation. By the latter we do not mean the total absence of sound or human contact but, rather, that such is either so rhythmic, mechanical, or out of context with the patient's usual set of expectancies that it's difficult to maintain an inner orientation as to time and place.

This is a common experience among those who remain in intensive care for prolonged periods. Here the constant, unchanging, around-the-clock vigilance of the hospital staff give little chance for discrimination between night and day. Sleep patterns may be disturbed, and perceptions upset as to the passage of time. Cardiac monitors, intravenous tubing, catheters, drains, and other assorted devices invading the body and capable of taking over virtually all physiological functions are terrifying in their intimations of physical discontinuity and loss. These experiences, in combination with the physical insult itself, may precipitate panic or even an acute, albeit transient, psychotic break.

CASE 57.   A 19-year-old male had been in a serious motorcycle accident in which, among other injuries, he had fractured his pelvis and legs. He was in the intensive care unit and in traction for more than a month. In the early stages he frequently believed himself to be driving a racing car that had crashed and caught on fire. He thought his traction device to be the car's safety harness that he had to undo to get out. In later months he clearly remembered these delusions and the problem he posed in his irrational and panicked efforts to escape.

Fortunately, episodes of this sort are not all that common and when they do occur are usually short-lived and without serious emotional sequelae. But while they last, they can pose a major management problem. As such reactions are usually paranoid in type, various life support systems may be pulled out and food and care refused, or the staff may be seen as the enemy engaged in a conspiracy against the patient himself, precipitating an apparently unaggravated assault. When such a psychosis does supervene, immediate tranquilization with one of the phenothiazide group is indicated (if not medically contraindicated) along with prompt psychiatric consultation.

Isolation represents a somewhat different state of affairs. Whether to protect others from exposure to infectious disease or to protect the patient because of deficient immunity, removing a teen-ager from peer contact creates its own set of problems. In addition, approaching the patient only in gown and mask magnifies his sense of being an outcast with something terribly wrong. Marked anger, depression, and withdrawal or, alternatively, acting out through elopement are understandable complications.

The adage "An ounce of prevention is worth a pound of cure" is particularly apt in any of these dissociative situations. Within the confines of reality, every effort should be made to promote verbal and human contact and relatedness to reality. In the recovery room or intensive care unit this means that biological ministrations should always be accompanied by talking to the patient in personal terms, rather than regarding him or her as simply an object of medical care. The purpose of the various life support systems should also be explained in a reassuring way. A radio or television playing at the bedside will also help. In isolation areas, telephones, closed-circuit television connecting the patient's room with the rest of the ward, definitive recreational and educational programs, and frequent visiting by family and ward staff are also all helpful adjuncts for minimizing the distancing effects of this experience.

RECURRENT HOSPITALIZATION FOR CHRONIC ILLNESS

Repeated Admissions. We have dwelled at some length on chronic illness, its meaning, and its management. But we would like to say yet a further word about those particular adolescents who must be admitted for relatively long and repeated hospitalizations and who spend a goodly part of their lives on the ward. Recurrent admissions seriously threaten the most important tasks of adolescence in establishing independence, peer relationships, and role definition. In order to be minimally disruptive, patients should be cared for by the same personnel on each admission insofar as is possible. These youths should also be granted maximum feasible freedom throughout their stay, with normal adolescent activities and frequent passes to the outside being provided to the degree that the condition permits. To these ends, teen-aged patients can be encouraged to wear street clothing while on the ward if they feel well enough, and to engage actively in schooling, recreation programs, and peer interaction.

Urogenital Anomalies.   We would also like to draw attention to another small group of chronically afflicted adolescents, usually (but not exclusively) males. This consists of those who require repeated or seriously disruptive genitourinary surgery for such congenital anomalies as extrophy, hypospadias, or ambiguous genitalia; or where ureteral obstruction or reflux has required the diversion of normal urinary pathways. In any of these situations concern is usually focused on the preservation of renal integrity and the restoration of normal architecture, with little thought and attention given to sexual function. Girls with parallel anomalies are usually prepared for such consequences as menstrual abnormalities and problems in bearing a child. But neither boys nor girls are ever given much chance to explore their worries and fears about sexual performance. Even though not sexually active, this is a matter of paramount importance to adolescents, and defects in sexual integrity can have profound effects upon body-image concepts and identity formation. Yet the questions that these adolescents invariably have about erection, ejaculation, intercourse, orgasm, and masturbation and the fears that they have about differences from normal peers are nearly always totally ignored.

CASE 58.   A 15-year-old biologically mature male had been born with extrophy of the bladder and penile epispadias. His present postsurgical appearance consisted of a short, stubby penis and multiple lower abdominal scars. When erect, his penis curved upward into a backward C and actually touched the abdominal wall. His ureters had been implanted into the sigmoid and the bladder removed. The youth could not imagine how he could ever expose himself to a female in this state, much less consummate the act of intercourse. In consequence, he planned never to marry and was unable to bring himself even to date. He also had problems among his peers in dealing with the fact that he could only void per rectum. He frequently stood with the other boys at the school urinal pretending to void in the normal way. Prior to the present admission for an annual review of his renal status, no one had ever talked to him of these things before. He was greatly relieved to be able to do so and indeed had much on his mind. At this point in time he was far more preoccupied with his inability to perform sexually or void in a normal way than he ever had been about the condition of his kidneys.

Inevitably, we find that these youths have rather extreme body-image distortions and severe anxiety about their genital deficiencies during the entire phase of adolescent development. Medical management requires alertness and sensitivity to these concerns and to the patient's singular need for consummate tact and privacy. One may need to be accepting of a reasonable amount of compensatory bravado as well. Intimate pre- and postoperative care should always be provided by a nurse, aide, or orderly of the same sex.

The youth will need to discuss even his most intimate concerns with the primary physician or consultant in adolescent medicine or psychiatry. Usually the youth will not volunteer his fears, and may even deny that they exist if asked only whether he has "anything on his mind." Instead, the situation should be directly appraised. The questioner should state that the patient is probably concerned about his or her sexuality and then proceed to review specific functional issues in detail.

The management of these youngsters is also a matter for the team planning conference. A patient's genital anomalies often create significant anxiety in the staff, who frequently handle their discomfiture by avoidance and denial or by tasteless and insensitive joking on rounds. Obviously, neither alternative has much to commend it. A more constructive approach should be taken.

Psychogenic Disease.   Certain chronic disorders with a significant psychological genesis sometimes require exceptions to the general rules of adolescent care. This is particularly true in cases of anorexia nervosa. In such cases, separation from home and family is often a definitive part of the therapeutic strategy, and hospitalization may be for psychological rather than purely medical needs. Furthermore, those ward activities, peer interactions, and free visitations that are to be encouraged for other patients may have to be restricted here in following the principles of behavior modification. It is particularly important that psychiatric and medical care be carefully coordinated and that all personnel maintain a unified front in supporting what may appear to be harsh and punitive measures.

PROFOUNDLY MUTILATING PROCEDURES

Probably nothing is more difficult or grievously experienced by all concerned than when a grossly mutilative surgical procedure must be performed upon a seemingly well youth. We shall address our remarks to what we are most familiar with—amputation for osteogenic sarcoma—but our management principles for youths undergoing this procedure may be directly extrapolated and applied to parallel situations as well.

Few medical circumstances are as difficult for the patient, parent, and staff to cope with than in the loss of a visible and integral part of the body. This is singularly true for osteogenic sarcoma. In the typical case, the youth has had relatively minimal and seemingly benign symptoms; when investigation reveals a malignancy, the only hope of survival is often through an immediate amputation. Not all youngsters thus afflicted are good candidates for resection and a prosthetic joint replacement alone. Matters that had heretofore been viewed in relatively calm and benign terms suddenly turn into a true crisis. Both parents and patient are exquisitely vulnerable to emotional collapse. A firm, well-planned, and highly supportive management approach is essential.

Although we have suggested always seeking the adolescent's willing and informed consent to surgery we exempt this situation from such a rule. No teen-ager is really able to consent freely to his own mutilation. The patient's narcissistic investment in physical normalcy and attractiveness virtually prohibits its voluntary acceptance.

Rather, we recommend that parents alone be told of the need for amputation as soon as a definitive diagnosis is made, and that they then be prepared to support this decision when it is time to tell their child. Best deferred until a relatively short time before surgery itself, the "announcement" should be delivered in *fait accompli* terms. Then no more than seventy-two hours should elapse before surgery. Even better, no more than one day. This provides just about the right length of time for working through feelings in the best way one can under the circumstances. If this period is too extended, the benefits of anticipatory grief rapidly drop off and anxiety escalates up the other side toward panic or unconstructive denial. Under no circumstances should the youth be taken to surgery in ignorance of what is to come. Such naive and denying (though often well-intentioned) actions will inevitably produce an extreme and untoward postoperative response, leaving the patient mistrustful, angry, and bereft in even more heightened terms than if he had been honestly prepared in advance. It can then be difficult to motivate the youth into taking an active and aggressive rehabilitational course.

A mature nurse or other staff member should be assigned to the patient on admission with the goal of establishing a primary transference relationship. This allows the youth who is psychologically available to begin to ventilate and work through feelings in advance of the surgery itself. But no patient should be pressured into verbalizing his fears. Rather, the staff must sensitively follow the youth's own lead. Another point to be kept in mind is that sometimes the adolescent may not feel able to talk as easily to the assigned professional as to another, and the ward care system needs to be flexible on this count.

In addition, parents will need their own support and should not be ignored out of preoccupation with the patient. The social worker and house staff officer, in concert with the surgeon, will be most often involved.

Precisely how the adolescent will respond following surgery is an individual matter, depending upon his premorbid personality, his particular developmental stage, and the adequacy of psychological preparation and ongoing support. But a certain amount of depression and mourning is inevitable and to be expected. One also frequently encounters denial of the full extent of permanent effects. While it is true that denial is often relatively ineffective, as well as dangerous when it postpones needed care, in this instance it beneficially serves to ward off excessive depression.

CASE 59. A 13-year-old girl had had a mid-thigh amputation of her left leg because of osteogenic sarcoma just one week before. Having rapidly and eagerly learned crutch walking, she was now up and about. She dealt with her loss primarily by the denial of any ultimate residual permanent effects upon her appearance and function, and anticipated that her prosthesis would recapitulate her lost extremity in the utmost detail. She did not plan to return to school until she was fully rehabilitated several months hence, at which time she believed that no one would be the wiser. Out of this denial the girl was able to pursue ambulation vigorously, avoid feeling too mutilated and devalued, and minimize fears of peer group abandonment. There would be time enough later on, after she had rescued her sense of self-esteem and personal integrity through compensation, for her to give up denial and come to grips with the reality of her new appearance and limitations.

Postoperative management of the mutilated youth is primarily geared at enabling the patient to become as mobile, independent, and self-managing as he or she can in the shortest period of time, and one should attempt to keep mourning or self-pity from moving too far toward despair. Physiotherapy, occupational and recreational therapy, rehabilitation medicine, and educational and peer group processes should all be introduced early in the convalescent course. Here, too, other adolescents who have had the same procedure and have successfully negotiated their own rehabilitation can be helpful models for positive identification and are often most willing to help. As an offshoot, this also beneficially serves the latter by enhancing their own sense of self-esteem in demonstrating just how well they have done. All possible modes that will help the patient regain function, resume maturational drives, resecure a sense of self-worth, and allay fears of rejection and abandonment should be introduced. He should not be viewed as crippled, nor should his parents and overidentifying staff members be allowed to be overprotective and solicitously perpetuate physical or emotional dependence. At times one may need to be quite harsh and firm on this point. For continued regression only robs the youth of his chance for personal growth and for a genuine adjustment to his altered self-perception.

SERIOUS ACCIDENTS

Serious accidents and their associated complications, such as burns, or orthopedic and neurological damage, represent the ultimate in disorganizing and overwhelming experiences for patient and parents alike. This situation involves all the problems already discussed, but in a highly exaggerated form. In addition to the sudden catastrophic interruption of a formerly healthy life, there are the further complications of prolonged hospitalization with profound immobilization and dependence, as well as very real possibilities for being permanently impaired.

During the acute phase, attentions are primarily directed at survival with the usual dynamic considerations of adolescence being temporarily put aside. Not until life is secured will it be appropriate to do much more than attempt to keep the patient in contact with moment-to-moment reality. But once stabilization is achieved and early convalescence begins, one must again promptly take up concerns for the restoration and preservation of emotional as well as biological health. This phase is almost always characterized by a severe reactive depression, with all its attendant grief, guilt, and anger. Not only is there the nature of the injury to contend with, but the causality of such trauma is often of such a futile and outrageous nature as to make these matters seem even worse.

CASE 60.   A 16-year-old boy who planned on an athletic career slid into home base during a high school baseball game. He impacted his head on the catcher's led guard and transected his cord at the neck with a resultant permanent quadriplegia.

CASE 61.   An 18-year-old youth, celebrating his engagement with a group of friends, was romping in a field. He decided to vault over an innocent-looking stone wall, only to plunge head first into an unexpected excavation on the other side. He became paraplegic.

CASE 62.   After a bitter argument with her parents, a 14-year-old girl decided to run away. She made a long rope from her bedsheets and blanket, as she lived in a sixth-floor apartment, and other than eloping from her window she thought she would be sure to get caught by her parents. She climbed about halfway down, but then slipped and fell the remaining three stories. She suffered severe and irreversible brain damage.

Frequently, post-traumatic reactive depressions are profound, and suicidal wishes are common at this time, rising from a sense of total helplessness, dependency, and despair. Sadly enough, these perceptions of a nearly overwhelming and desperate loss often bear a good measure of truth.

CASE 63.   A healthy 14-year-old boy was standing on a curb talking with a friend. A nearby delivery truck backed up unexpectedly, hitting them both. The friend was killed and the boy suffered serious injury to his brain. Subsequently he became mute, partially spastic, and unable to tend to himself. He had a rather blank and drooling expression and walked with a shuffling, slow gait. He was a sad image of his former self. Nonetheless, he developed modes of nonverbal communication with his family. In his own fashion he made it very clear to his parents that they were to put away all pictures of him as he had been and all mirrors were to be covered or taken down. It was quite obvious that the boy was fully aware of all that he had lost.

In managing such patients, the initial psychotherapeutic responsibility rests with the primary physician and floor nurse. For it is they who can best provide support and understanding and who can best help the youth to discriminate between reality and distorted fantasy in coming to terms with his true state. A mental health professional is also necessary, not only to support and direct the primary caring personnel, but also to institute long-term psychotherapeutic measures with the patient himself. But at no point should the primary physician abdicate his ongoing role, and he should continue to talk with the patient for a few minutes each day and for longer periods two or three times a week, even when a psychotherapist is involved.

Yet another problem is the monumental task of coordinating the functions of all who are involved. Patients who have sustained serious injuries to a number of organ systems inevitably require the services of a host of specialists and technicians. It is no easy matter to integrate everything into an orderly program of care. Repeated coordinating conferences will be needed to accomplish this goal, with the primary physician and team nurse firmly in charge.

From another perspective, one cannot overlook the effects of caring for the seriously ill and injured upon the staff itself, particularly that burden placed upon nursing personnel. First is the problem of taking care of a physically large but helpless youth who needs constant and vigilant attention. This is tiresome and tedious work. In addition, the adolescent who is forced into an infantilized state in both physical and emotional terms can be difficult indeed. When the situation is prolonged, unavoidable annoyance or outright anger at a patient's continued regressive and demanding behavior can undermine even the best of therapeutic plans. This is most apt to occur when the staff's views about just how cooperative, stoic, or good-naturedly acquiescent the adolescent ought to be are substantially at variance with the true state of affairs. It is sometimes only too tempting for professionals to take the path of least resistance in dealing with these feelings by avoiding contact with the patient or handing over care to others.

Obviously, such defensive maneuvers only add to the difficulties and serve everyone poorly. The potential for this type of "acting out" by professionals needs to be honestly recognized and taken up in the team conference, where affected staff members can be given every support. Those in distress may then be able to return to their patients with some degree of equanimity—even in the face of provocative hostility, negativism, or outright nastiness. We do not wish to imply that the staff need always be smilingly uncritical or benignly accepting of this type of behavior. They can, and indeed should, convey to the patient that he or she is expected to do better, but they must also patiently accept the fact that this may take some time. Continued sensitivity to the terrible insult that the adolescent has experienced, and to the very real threat that this situation poses to her or his ever again being whole, will help engender a sense of tolerance and forbearance.

In the opposite vein, staff members sometimes also become depressed by their patient's poor outlook. If anger and resentment is one set of feelings they must contend with, no less is the problem of countertransference when one has to deal with a youth whose life chances seem to have been destroyed. It can be singularly difficult to avoid sharing the depression of an adolescent who is newly paraplegic, devastatingly scarred, or permanently handicapped in some other profound way—and this usually from a mindless and stupid cause. Here, too, answers will best be found through problem-solving conferences, and it is most important that staff be willing to discuss these feelings openly and not try to suppress or deny what is very human and real.

Although we espouse continuity in the caring for any particular youth, we also urge that the burden of managing consecutive severely damaged patients be shared and not always left solely to those who seem to be emotionally strongest. Any staff member who has been providing continuous care to the devastatingly ill needs at least a brief break and a temporary shift to tending for those with more optimistic prospects.

Many of these adolescents face months of hospitalization, multiple operations, and protracted rehabilitation. It is probably inevitable that normal development will in some measure be set back.

CASE 64.   A 20-year-old male had been in a serious automobile accident three years before. Multiple fractures and soft tissue injuries had rather persistently threatened his life and kept him in and out of the hospital for the better part of two years. Further, he had been unable to return to school or to graduate with his class. He lived some distance from the hospital and had gradually lost contact with his friends. Prior to this time he had been a vigorous and outgoing teen-ager, socially adept, had done well in his classes, and had planned on some sort of a professional career. But now, although he had fully recovered and had been essentially well for a year, he was no longer interested in his former pursuits, felt anxious when away from his home, and was unable to reintegrate successfully with his peers or to begin to date again. He was both aware of and distressed by these symptoms and had finally come to request psychiatric help.

To minimize the effects illustrated in the above case, every effort is needed to assist such youths to be autonomous as soon as they can and to return to their normal affairs and usual environment with all reasonable dispatch. This will mean seeing to it that they receive the benefits of every technical advance in providing them with optimum mobility, psychotherapeutic support, vocational training, and congress with normal as well as similarly afflicted peers.

RENAL DIALYSIS AND TRANSPLANTS

Dialysis.   The demands of chronic dialysis and its associated stringent dietary limitations are particularly stressful for the adolescent. These restrictions are in direct opposition to all the maturational drives of these years. Enforced continued dependence upon others (and the dialysis machine as well), decreased freedom and mobility, interruption of family life, curtailment in peer socialization, and frequent absences from school collectively impose a burden of enormous magnitude. However great the temptation to rebel and resist these restricting forces may be, this is firmly and irrevocably constrained by the fact that to refuse to comply means death. In our estimate these are matters that strongly mitigate against these youngsters ever being able to tolerate and effectively cope with a chronic dialysis program for much more than six months. Hence every effort to provide them with a kidney transplant as early as possible should be made. It is difficult to establish priorities between one group and another in relation to need where cadaver kidneys are concerned. We can but hope that those who make decisions in these matters will take the singular stresses of adolescence into good account.

The management goal for these youths is, as for others, to attempt to provide as close an approximation to a normal life style as is possible. To this end, dialysis should be carried out during the night, either in hospital or home. Daytime procedures, whether during school or weekend hours, are obviously far more disruptive.

It should also be recognized that depression is universally present early in the course and, with the passage of time, often advances into conscious or unconscious suicidal acting out. This may be manifest by dietary noncompliance and the ignoring of other vital aspects of therapy. The result can be repeated crisis hospitalizations as well as considerable conflict and confrontation between the patient and those adults who are responsible for his care. Denial may also be operative, to the youth's similar detriment, through failing to comply with the treatment regimen or through the invocation of some other form of impulsive and inappropriate behavior.

CASE 65. A 17-year-old youth with chronic renal disease (Alport's syndrome) was rapidly approaching serious kidney failure. He was well aware of all that this meant as an older sister had been similarly ill and had undergone dialysis and then transplant some five years before. Although she had done well and was still living, she had an unattractive Cushingoid appearance due to continuing steroid therapy. Hypochondriacal by nature, she unendingly complained about her health as well. In addition, his sister's total course had been studded with horrendous complications and heroic measures. When the youth was told of his own impending need, he refused to believe that this was true; and, to prove to the contrary, he eloped with his girlfriend and took off for an indefinite transcontinental tour. However, his increasing debility forced him to return several weeks later and he finally accepted the necessity of dialysis. Unfortunately, in this instance a cadaver kidney is necessary and the boy is of an unusual type. It will be some time before a suitable donor can be found. His girlfriend, not knowing of his illness before or even of his still tender age, had the marriage annulled. The patient is now markedly depressed and continues to require close psychiatric supervision and care.

However, there is one meager advantage in working with these younsters: they are often quite well known to the staff consequent to the many years of their disease and past admissions. Thus there should be ample time to develop a solid basis for a collaborative and mutually trusting relationship well in advance of instituting these difficult therapies. This may make matters a little easier for all concerned.

Transplantation. Since much study has been given to the implications of organ transplant itself, we do not propose to discuss them here except for two points about this procedure as it applies to youth. First, considerable distortion of exactly what will happen and what to expect inevitably occurs, and special efforts will be needed to encourage and reinforce continued reality-based perceptions. Second, there is a tendency for teen-aged transplant recipients to view this procedure as a total cure and to believe that if they survive they will need no further care. Few are prepared for the iatrogenically induced moon-faced appearance, intensification of acne, and generalized obesity that they must endure as a consequence of steroid therapy and immunosuppression. Nor are they always aware of the possiblility of periodic rejection threats that may recur from time to time and the positive things that can be done. While we do not wish to suggest that one should paint a bleak and frightening picture of what is to come, a rational amount of preoperative honesty will help keep the youth from having totally unrealistic expectations about just how normal and free of medical supervision he will be. To be unprepared for significant distortions in physical appearance and to be ignorant of the continued need for close supervision will make it much more difficult for normally narcissistic and emancipating adolescents to cope with these matters when they do arise. Too often such preparation is overlooked. No greater reward can accrue to a medical staff than to give life to a child or adolescent who was formerly doomed to dialysis or death. It is easy to avoid discussing those matters that will dilute and detract from the perfection of this gift.

MENTAL RETARDATION

The youth who is mentally retarded will be admitted to the hospital for all the same reasons as any other person of his or her age. This group is perhaps even more subject to infectious illness than others and certainly more apt to be afflicted with epilepsy, cerebral palsy, and congenital heart disease. Yet the discordance between a retarded youth's physical development and his intellectual capacity often makes it difficult for him to fit into the hospital milieu at all. Special approaches are needed.

The most important first step is for the ward staff to be aware that the patient is in fact retarded. While this may seem to be an obvious statement, it is not unusual for a retarded youth to arrive on the floor with no one aware of his state. And it may not be obvious right away. Many are good-looking youngsters with normal physical development. This is certainly a matter that the staff should be apprised of in advance, or at the very least no later than at the time of the admitting history and physical examination.

The severely affected adolescent—who is virtually noncommunicating, extremely limited in his capacity, and often suffering from a profound concomitant retardation in his physical size—is a far different problem than the one who is educable or trainable and has a statural and biological maturity more or less commensurate with his age. The former group are generally best managed if placed with younger children or even toddlers; while physically well-developed youths will probably be most comfortably managed on the adolescent ward, even if their behavioral level is comparable to those of much younger years. Certainly placement of this group should depend solely on development and function rather than age, even though this may cause consternation in the admitting office or to some members of the staff.

In managing those retarded youths who are at an educable or trainable level (and who will undoubtedly be on the adolescent ward), it is essential to realize that they are often painfully aware of their deficiencies and of being "stupid" and "dumb." Emotionally and affectively, they have all the same feelings and instinctive drives as do their nonimpaired peers and need the acceptance and affection of others and opportunities for gaining self-esteem just as much as does anyone else. But these teen-agers will be handicapped by concreteness of thought, immature behavior, impulse difficulties, sexual confusion, and the like.

Retarded individuals can be deeply hurt by teasing and deprecating remarks. They also tend to be very sensitive about being talked down to in a condescending or infantile way. Each of these patients will require gentleness, compassion, and understanding coupled with a keen sensitivity to the enormous gap that exists between the fullness of their emotional feelings and self-awareness in contrast to their diminished and limited capacity to cope effectively. In managing these youths it is important to use the same basic approach as to any other patient on the ward, with the addition of special cognitive supports. Even significantly impaired adolescents can understand what is going on to some degree, and they should be frequently told why they are in the hospital, what is going to be done to make them well, and what they must do to help.

As most of these youngsters are already distressed by separation from home and disruption of their normal routines, they tend to arrive on the ward in a highly frightened and retreating state. To impose unexpected medical care arbitrarily only makes matters worse. A few minutes spent in advance preparation through simplified explanation and demonstration will more than pay off in increased cooperation and will go a long way in helping to avoid a panic reaction by the patient.

Perhaps the major problem in managing retarded youth rests in their impulsive and confused behavior. Such adolescents often tend to mix up a variety of matters such as sexual feelings and aggressive impulses. Staff also become confused by their own expectations in light of the patient's physical size and biological maturity. Thus, when a retarded youth fails to understand and comply with what he is told, this may be misperceived as adolescent rebellion and recalcitrance. Too, childlike behavior may not be so readily acceptable from one who is reproductively mature.

CASE 66.   A moderately retarded but physically well-developed 14-year-old boy was admitted for repair of congenital heart disease. His medical and surgical course was benign and he did well throughout his stay. However, he became somewhat of a problem as he persistently hugged and kissed everyone on the ward, including patients, visitors, and members of the ward staff. The problem was not so much his behavior alone, but this in contrast to his physical size. Although the boy's actions clearly consisted of infantile gestures, the adults on the ward could not help their own discomfiture over the apparent inappropriateness of his behavior in light of his genital maturity; nor could they divest themselves of conditioned expectations and accept the clear discrepancy between the youth's physical and mental state. Had the patient been but a toddler of three or four, which was in fact not far from his true capacity, similar attentions would have caused little distress.

Behavioral problems of retarded youths are best met by having a highly consistent and predictable environment, firm continuity in caring personnel, and a structured schedule. Educational, occupational, and recreational staff can be of particular help; their assistance should be enlisted early and maintained throughout the patient's stay.

PREGNANCY AND ABORTION

Hospitalization for delivery or abortion is but a small part of the totality of events surrounding a teen-ager's pregnancy. And the primary responsibility rests largely with those who are helping the girl with her long-range care and future plans. We do not intend to address the concerns of such comprehensive services here. Nevertheless, it is germane to say a few words about managing these adolescents when they are on the ward. As we noted in discussing the hospital setting, this is one exception to the rule of admitting all teen-agers to the same floor. If the girl plans on keeping her baby and establishing her own home, she has in some measure elected to function as an adult insofar as she can, and her primary role is that of a young mother. In this instance her admission to the obstetrical floor with other new mothers is most appropriate. It is essential, of course, that those who are providing her out-patient care continue to visit and give her support while on the ward and to provide continuity between her pre- and postnatal periods.

There may, however, be some exceptions to this admitting policy. While few unmarried pregnant adolescents today go to term with the view of surrendering their children for adoption, some still do. These teen-agers see themselves as not yet ready to assume the responsibility of parenthood and wish to return to the business of their own growing up. In this instance they are still functioning as adolescents and one may well wish to admit them to the adolescent ward.

More debate exists over abortions. Two arguments obtain here. The first states that an adolescent who is terminating her pregnancy, with all its emotional strain, may be more comfortable and will obtain better support and acceptance on the abortion ward; and that the condition rather than age should be the determining factor. On the other hand, one may also validly argue that this event should be handled as simply another surgical procedure in a teen-ager with admission to the adolescent floor. This latter perspective is particularly pertinent where the hospital has but a single obstetrical and gynecological ward and where the patient admitted here for abortion will be surrounded by those who are delivering as well.

In actual practice both methods can work well; and in this instance, as elsewhere, a flexible approach should be applied. The adolescent herself is usually mature enough to decide which ward she would prefer, and the hospital should be open-minded enough to allow her choice. If she is not mature enough to come to a decision on her own, she probably is sufficiently young as to do better with her agemates. This is most true for those of 11, 12, and 13 years, as these girls often have little sense of relatedness to their gravid condition.

It should also be noted that, as far as can be determined, adolescents bear no greater or lesser potential for permanent psychological harm from abortion than do older females. An emotionally healthy girl who has freely made this decision will have few long-term sequelae, although she will undoubtedly have a quite normal period of mourning and grief. Those who have preexisting emotional difficulties or who have been forced into an abortion against their own inner feelings are the ones who are at significant risk and may have major problems later on. Some adolescents have serious delayed depressive reactions with suicidal ideation about six months after the procedure itself. Others may seek to undo their loss by becoming pregnant again.

In any event, it is important that there be firm lines of communication between not only obstetrical and adolescent medical staff but also in-patient services and out-patient care. Pregnancy in an unwed adolescent often involves many professionals, including a primary physician, obstetrician, consultant psychiatrist, out-patient nurse, social worker, and special education program personnel, as well as the entire ward staff. In this situation alertness is needed lest major coordination breakdowns occur.

Confidentiality is an important matter in abortion and out-of-wedlock delivery. These procedures are usually carried out under highly private circumstances. In some instances this may even be without the knowledge of the girl's parents. While we generally believe that teen-agers are best served if they have the support of their families at this time, we pragmatically accept the fact that parental involvement may not always be possible or even wise. It is also incontrovertible that some adolescents are indeed sufficiently mature as to be able to give a valid and informed consent, and thus are entitled to the constitutional right of privacy and to receive confidential care on their own. These views are becoming confirmed in the statutory provisions of an increasing number of states (see chapter 13). Hospitals must consider methods of protecting these confidences and of keeping the patient's record from unauthorized view.

No matter what ward the pregnant adolescent is admitted to and whatever her course, the most critical aspect of care is to make her hospitalization as positive an experience as possible. This depends largely on staff attitudes. All must be able to treat the patient, her pregnancy, and her abortion in a nonjudgmental and nonpunitive way. Anyone who cannot refrain from directly or indirectly attempting to impose his or her own preferential views has no business caring for these young women. It is for the patient herself (and her family when involved) to deal with moral issues and conflicts. The role of the staff is to help the girl make the best—or "least worse"—decision that she can in light of her own beliefs and needs; and then to support her in carrying it out. These adolescents all suffer their own confusions, ambivalences, and pangs of guilt, and are hardly benefited by having these matters further aggravated and burdened by the biases of others. This is just as applicable to the professional who expresses displeasure at a 14-year-old for going to term and keeping her child rather than having an abortion and thereby "ruining her life," as it is to the one who views sex before marriage as an immoral act or regards abortion as a truly cardinal sin. We do not dispute the right of a professional to hold such personal views, but we are firm in our position that these must not be visited upon the patient who is under his or her charge. Empathetic, reasoned, and rational support is what the girl needs most while in search of her own most responsible decision.

SUICIDAL THREATS AND ATTEMPTS

Suicidal ideation and acting out are not at all uncommon in adolescence. In the hospital setting, concepts of terminating one's own life are most often associated with reactive depressions following serious illness or surgery with some form of permanent loss. We have already noted this phenomenon to occur with some regularity in the early convalescent stage of those with traumatic para- or quadriplegias and, as a somewhat later event, in the course of long-term renal hemodialysis.

Expression of a suicidal wish may occasionally complicate a considerably less dire hospitalization. This is most often associated with a recent object loss unrelated to the illness itself, possibly quite unknown to the staff. The youth who has just broken off with a girl- or boyfriend, has suffered a parental death, separation, or divorce, or in some other way has had a meaningful relationship newly terminated must be considered vulnerable.

In other instances an actual suicidal attempt will be the cause for admission to the ward, as occasioned by a self-inflicted wound or intentional drug overdose. Not infrequently such an act will have been precipitated by the severance of a romance or a bitter family argument, with the youth carrying out the suicidal gesture as both a punishment to those he or she is angry with and as a cry for help. Most frequently seen are adolescent girls who have superficially slashed their wrists or taken a number of aspirin or minor tranquilizers. The adolescent would-be suicide has been well characterized by Teicher.

Some accidents also are suicidal at heart, and such an underlying motivation should be looked for when the incident seems to have no rational cause and seems more than simple miscalculation. It may well be an operative factor among young males who crash into roadside abutments or trees while driving alone. A similar theory applies to those who are accident prone.

CASE 67. Within one year, a 14-year-old boy "accidentally" sprained his ankle in basketball, cut his hand quite badly on some glass, was beaten up by a neighborhood gang, had a light bulb "explode" in his eye, broke a finger playing baseball, got hit by a truck while crossing a road, underwent three negative laparotomies in four months' time for abdominal pain, and was in an automobile accident while riding in the passenger's seat. Although this last episode appeared to exonerate the youth from any complicity, one is convinced that he somehow still had a hand in it. He was well known to both adolescent medicine and psychiatry as being deeply disturbed, and it was quite clear that his accidents were all prompted both by unconscious suicidal wishes and by a desire for the protective insulation of the hospital to fend off his own self-destructive impulses.

Suicidal behavior may derive from an even more profoundly depressed and psychopathological state or a true psychosis. In these instances, suicidal wishes bear a real likelihood of being carried out. A careful history should always be obtained from any youngster who seems singularly depressed. There is probably no simpler method of finding out than by asking the patient directly. As most adolescents are very frightened by inner impulses to end their lives, they will often willingly admit them out of a genuine desire for help. Although such information is rarely volunteered, simply asking the youth in a straightforward manner whether she or he has ever considered suicide will almost always produce an honest response. It is not necessary to be circuitous in approach. Nor need one fear that a nonsuicidal youngster will be offended by such an intimate inquiry.

Regardless of the seeming genesis or method of presentation, *any* adolescent who expresses suicidal thoughts or makes a suicidal attempt should *always* be taken seriously. Even if it seems to be a "safe" and passing gesture (rather than a true attempt), a thorough assessment of the degree of risk and the advisability of keeping the patient on the open ward should be carried out by the liaison psychiatrist as soon as possible. In the interim, the youth should be engaged in relating to others as much as possible during daytime hours and should always be kept in view at night.

Not all adolescents who express suicidal thoughts, or even all those who make a suicidal attempt, require transfer to a locked psychiatric ward. This is probably only necessary for a small number of the most depressed who are unable to establish positive affective relationships with the staff. Others can be quite effectively maintained on the medical ward throughout their stay, and may even benefit by being there. The well-run and well-supervised adolescent floor is by its very nature a psychotherapeutic milieu and a highly protective environment, even though its primary intent is to render medical care. Staff need not panic for fear that a youth whom psychiatry deems safe to remain on the ward will immediately harm himself as long as reasonable vigilance, continued affective contact, and a relatively structured program are maintained.

Any teen-ager who has indicated that he has thoughts of terminating his life is in deep emotional pain, and some sort of assistance is mandatory. For those remaining on the adolescent medical ward, this will vary from simple support and ventilation by medical personnel—as may be most appropriate for the reactively depressed in the face of a serious reality-based medical state—to definitive psychotherapy for those with a preexisting psychological problem. Again, these decisions rest upon careful and individualized planning between all involved under the guidance of the liaison mental health professional.

PSYCHOTIC BREAKS

Adolescence is one of the first major periods in life in which latent psychotic vulnerabilities may emerge. The formative stresses of these years, in combination with the added strain and confusion posed by serious medical illness, may pinpoint hospitalization as the force tipping the precarious balances of the borderline schizophrenic toward decompensation.

CASE 68. A 16-year-old boy was admitted for a spontaneous pneumothorax following a vigorous basketball practice. He was successfully treated by chest suction alone and went home in less than a week. He tolerated this admission well, although he did seem a little remote. His history revealed that he had been briefly hospitalized three years before, following a suicidal threat over feelings of rejection by a favored teacher at school. Subsequently, matters had seemed to calm down and he was doing relatively well.

Several months after his initial hospitalization the pneumothorax recurred and he was readmitted for a thoracotomy and pleural scarification, a much more extensive and threatening procedure. Medically he did well, but during convalescence it was noted that he often had a peculiar, staring look on his face and that he seemed increasingly out of touch with what was going on. He gradually became more and more agitated over when he could leave and began to accuse the staff of keeping him against his will for their own ill-defined purposes, while at the same time developing an inordinate and frequently expressed crush on a recreation worker on the ward. One day, after she firmly rejected his advances, he suddenly grabbed a kitchen knife, abortively threatened a nurse, and then climbed to a window to jump. Ultimately he was coaxed down. Now clearly out of contact with reality, he was quickly transferred to a locked ward. He has now been followed for three additional years. Although medically well, he continues to be a very disturbed youth and is maintained in a highly structured day-care program while living at home.

Obviously a full-blown acute psychotic episode such as demonstrated by this case represents an unmistakable psychiatric emergency requiring immediate intervention. However, had greater note been taken of his earlier problem and had therapy been instituted sooner, it might have been possible to avoid this crisis altogether. As we have consistently noted, there are almost always clues in the past history if looked for. When one is aware that a particular adolescent is at risk, prevention of a florid break then becomes a reasonable possibility. These measures consist of early and adequate medication for escalating anxiety (primarily with phenothiazides), supportive psychotherapy, and a highly programmed day. Usually somewhat eccentric, such adolescents are likely to be "loners" and may be difficult to handle at times, but they will generally respond quite well to an organized and consistent approach.

Psychotic youngsters should not be confused with those who are disturbed because of their medical state. The thinking disorder of true schizophrenia is quite different from the transient delusions and hallucinations of delirium, cognitive deprivation, or serious illness. In these latter instances there are no historical suggestions of emotional disease and the medical condition obviously contributes to the patient's mental state.

Occasionally, the adolescent medical ward will be faced with the need to care for a known psychotic adolescent. Such youths are as subject to illness and injury as anybody else. It is particularly important to enlist the help of the patient's outside therapist in both visiting and planning care. This provides essential knowledge to the staff and support to the youth in a strange setting, making for a far smoother course. Here, too, the use of psychotropic medication and a structured program is beneficial. In this instance, as in all others, life-preserving medical and surgical interventions always come first. For one fact is quite certain: effective psychiatric treatment and emotional support can take place only if the patient survives.

chapter eleven

Neurological and Orthopedic Handicaps

by Leon Greenspan, M.D.

The purpose of this chapter is to indicate some of the emotional and social problems of teen-agers hospitalized in a rehabilitation center. The adolescent who is disabled may have had a number of prior admissions or this may be his first time. The former situation includes those youngsters who have a variety of congenital abnormalities such as cerebral palsy, spina bifida manifesta with paraparesis and bowel and bladder incontinence, spinal atrophy, and progressive muscular dystrophy. These individuals have usually been hospitalized periodically throughout childhood for such matters as evaluation, rehabilitation, and orthopedic, urologic, or plastic surgery as the need arose. In the second instance we are primarily dealing with post-traumatic brain or cord injury, cerebrovascular accidents, and amputations—either traumatic or surgical consequent to malignancy. In any case, the length of stay is measured in months in contrast to the days or weeks of an acute hospital admission.

Dr. Leon Greenspan is Director of the Children's Division, Institute for Rehabilitation Medicine, New York University Medical Center, and Professor of Clinical Rehabilitation Medicine at New York University School of Medicine. We are pleased to be able to round out this book with this chapter by Dr. Greenspan. His extensive experience with the rehabilitation of the orthopedically and neurologically handicapped young is admirably reflected in this description of the world of the adolescent who is disabled. We suggest that the dynamic considerations and management approaches offered elsewhere are equally applicable here. But we would also like to stress the need to develop a balanced, structured, and meaningful day replete with education, recreation, discipline, responsibility, and contributing tasks for those teen-agers who are to be hospitalized for extended periods of time. Long-term in-patient care of the adolescent is a somewhat different matter than that for those who will have but a brief stay, requiring more attention to providing a milieu that allows for the resumption of personal growth in all its dimensions insofar as the condition permits.—A.D.H.

But, before dealing with specifics, it is necessary to define *rehabilitation medicine*. This is the phase of health care that is involved with the total needs of the disabled individual. The goal is to achieve maximum function and the restoration of all abilities to a degree that is both possible and realistic. It is a management program with the term *management* used in the context described by Bax and MacKeith. "Treatment involves measures aimed at curing or improving a disorder or disability. Management involves doing all that is humanly, medically possible to ease the difficulties and make life more rewarding for the patient, often multiply handicapped, and his family. Management is the continuing totality of all treatment of all the patient's dimensions, somatic, intellectual, emotional and social." With this orientation the reader will better understand the approach of the author, a pediatrician and a physiatrist.

It should also be noted that I do not believe in a "psychology" peculiar to disabled adolescents; but, rather, that these young people will have more overt and forceful expressions of their normal developmental conflicts. Handicapped teen-agers are intensely concerned with body image, peer acceptance, independence from parents, self-acceptance, and achievement. They are, however, much more prone to anger, depression, hostility, and mourning, and have the right to these feelings. The adolescent who is a quadriplegic, whatever the cause, has to undergo numerous indignities; turning of the body, dressing and undressing assistance, and management of bowel and bladder incontinence. They will be angry with parents for bringing them into the world as disabled individuals; angry with siblings for their sometimes limited and indifferent involvement; angry with peers because of avoidance; angry with the hospital staff who have not communicated with them as to what has been done, what is being done, and what lies ahead in the future; and angry at themselves for what they are. In addition to these reactions, there are others that must be considered in the rehabilitation process.

The Attitude of Parents. How parents feel about them is particularly important for adolescents with congenital disabilities. For this will have colored parent-child interactions from the beginning. The patient may be seen by the mother and father as indicative of their inability to bear a normal offspring, prompting guilt or feelings of inadequacy. Parents of a child with acquired defects also experience guilt feelings out of believing that they were not vigilant enough, or otherwise have failed in their nurturing role. The relationships between the parents and other members of the family are also important. The presence of a seriously handicapped youngster sometimes contributes significantly to intra-marital strife; or may result in either favoritism or the ignoring of other siblings, fostering jealousy. The degree to which the parents, and indeed the entire family, can come to accept the disability and deal with it in positive and loving terms will also strongly influence the patient's own ability to adapt constructively during adolescence and to pursue his own independence and identity in the best way he can.

Unfortunately, these youngsters are generally either overindulged and overprotected or, alternatively, neglected and rejected during their early years. Easson has noted that a child born with a congenital defect has to face not only the physical effects but also the emotional reactions of his family, which may be even more crippling to his total emotional and physical growth than the specific disability itself. The child who is disabled may consequently arrive at his teen years feeling that he is evil and unlovable, a person "who only a mother can love." Or he may be so infantilized and overprotected as to be unable to develop any meaningful autonomy at all, even if physically capable.

With the arrival of adolescence, parents also develop new concerns. As one mother of a brain-damaged youth stated so well, "What am I to do? He is maturing physically but not intellectually." Another parent of an adolescent boy with spina bifida manifesta said that as long as he was in his special class at school or in a rehabilitation program he was fine. But when he left he was in another world that was neither accepting of him nor he of it. At times he became extremely depressed in spite of all that his parents were trying to do for him.

Males with congenital disabilities may have problems in gender identification. In normal developmental processes, the more secure a boy is in his relationship with his father, the readier he is to enter manhood. Unfortunately, this relationship is often lacking for a child whose condition has associated bowel and bladder incontinence and requires help with dressing and bathing well beyond infancy. For it has usually fallen to the mother to tend to these intimate needs. Since these matters are a continuing and constant problem in those with spina bifida manifesta, dependence upon the mother persists for many years and the father's role is minimized. In contrast, girls with a similar disability can relate effectively to their mothers and hence come to accept womanhood with greater ease.

Personality Traits.   The quality of participation of an adolescent in a rehabilitation program will also be dependent to a certain degree upon the personality type of the individual. Some adolescents may be self-directed and strong willed, boding well for their course. An example is a young lady who became paraplegic as the result of a car accident. Prior to this expisode she was an excellent student with a bright future. Of course she was angry, sullen, and depressed at the onset of her rehabilitation program. But she worked "like a beaver" and rapidly became independent in all activities of daily living; she returned to her high school on a full program, was graduated with honors, and went on to college away from home. Today she is a productive professional person. Another adolescent who had congenital cerebral palsy, athetoid type, once said that if he were not "aggressive and self-directed" he would never have accomplished what he had.

It should be noted, however, that even a highly motivated adolescent with an acquired disability may not be willing to participate in an active rehabilitation program until after a period of mourning and adaptation. This was the situation with a 17-year-old male who became paraplegic as the result of an accident. He had been an outstanding football player. Not only he, but also his father and friends saw him as a future All-American and a star professional. Both the young man and his family, particularly the father, required considerable supportive therapy in dealing with this loss before he could mobilize and make use of his other assets, though the physical retained importance in his activities of daily living.

The adolescent who is a conforming and adaptive person usually also adjusts well in a rehabilitation center. But those who tend to be passive and submissive, who are followers and dependent upon authority, often present problems in adjusting to and participating in a program. The alienated and angry youth who has no true sense of identity, is negative about all that he does, and performs poorly in school is also one who poses difficulties. An example of the latter is the 18-year-old post-traumatic quadriplegic who was intellectually bright but never cared for school and was an underachiever. Prior to his accident he had been about to "drop out of school and be a bum." During his inpatient stay he was continuously depressed and uncommunicative. He had no interest in the program, nor in life itself. As far as he was concerned, if he could not have the physical use of his body no one could be of any help. Although he was intelligent he could not see himself as a useful person. This was his attitude before his accident and the accident only potentiated his preexisting feelings. In consequence, he would not accept any form of therapy.

The Specific Disability.   While it is not possible to discuss all the disabilities that would require rehabilitation during the adolescent years, the following are among the most common and serve to point out the spectrum of problems that confront these youngsters. *Cerebral palsy* may be either congenital or acquired. The former is the result of brain injury occurring from the time of conception through the perinatal period and the latter is caused by permanent central nervous system damage from meningitis, encephalitis, trauma, cerebrovascular accidents, and the like anytime thereafter. Specifically, cerebral palsy is a stable, nonprogressive neurological disorder of movement, posture, and coordination. One must keep in mind, however, that the motor deficit is only a part of the total picture and a variety of associated problems also must be taken into consideration. Seizures, sensory deficits, speech and language problems, behavioral and emotional aberrations, social and vocational adjustment, and, most important, learning disabilities are all part of this picture as well. The inability to communicate, as is the situation with an adolescent who has athetosis (and is usually of at least average intelligence), is frustrating indeed and often manifests itself in anger, bitterness, and emotional lability. The motor disability does not permit him to become independent; he must continue to require assistance from someone else in many activities of daily living. One teen-aged girl with this type of dysfunction said she wished she could find a man who is also disabled—but not to the degree that he would not be able to take care of her.

Spina bifida manifesta often results in motor weakness and sensory loss below the level of the lesion, together with bowel and bladder incontinence. Usual adolescent concerns for attractiveness and normalcy become exaggerated and frustrated. Not only do these teen-agers look different because of their motor disabilities, but they sometimes have great difficulty contending with the odors associated with bowel and bladder incontinence.

While males can be fitted with an appropriate urinary collecting device, female anatomy makes this matter infinitely more difficult for the girl. If not required earlier to control bladder infections and deteriorating renal function, a urinary diversional procedure such as an ileal conduit (Bricker procedure) can be carried out for purposes of improved hygiene. But, in and of itself, this step further alters normal biological function and may pose additional stress for body-image concepts. Therefore, before such a procedure, the patient must be fully aware of what is going to be done, why, and what it will look like. Further, she should be fully consenting and not feel unwilling victim or pawn to the decisions of others imposed upon her. If these steps are not taken, the teen-aged girl may well come to regard the conduit stoma on her abdominal wall as something ugly and feel even more devalued than she did before. She must also learn how to take care of the stoma and how to apply the collecting bag, developing a sense of confidence in self-management. The advantages of such a procedure are that there is no longer a need for diapers or pads, no smell, and no danger of an accident or skin breakdown.

Intermittent catheterization has recently been introduced as an alternative method of lessening residual urine and dribbling. This is being used in both males and females whose incontinence is due to the above lesion or who have a cord injury. With proper preparation, guidance, and encouragement it is possible for the patient to perform catheterization unassisted.

It should be noted here that some adolescents with spina bifida manifesta not only have the deficits noted above but also have the sequelae of brain damage resulting from the frequently associated hydrocephalus. This, of course, introduces yet another set of complications that must be dealt with, adding mental retardation to the picture.

A word should be said about sexuality in this condition or, indeed, for any youth with a spinal cord lesion that interferes with the innervation of the genital area or the motor functions associated with coitus. The female has normal or even precocious sexual development. In most instances she has a normal menarche, is fertile, and can and does view herself as a complete woman. The male, however, is not that fortunate. Although he does develop secondary sex characteristics, he views his incontinent penis as an incompetent one.*

The adolescent with *progressive muscular dystrophy*, Duchenne type—the most malignant form—is wheelchair bound, severely disabled with marked scoliosis and muscle weakness. He is dependent in all activities of daily living and faces a curtailed life span. Such youths are fully aware of their disability and the final outcome. Although they do not talk about an early death, they appear to accept it as inevitable. However, they want to be given all necessary assistance to function as long as possible and to have the opportunity to go to school, to join in activities with their peers, and to have as enriched a quality of life as is possible. One such adolescent said that his similarly afflicted brothers died because they gave up. He himself was not going to give up and wanted all possible therapeutic steps taken. In testimony to what can be achieved, a number of adolescents with progressive dystrophy have gone to college and had a number of vocationally productive years.

Reactions to the Rehabilitation Program.   Upon arrival at a rehabilitation program the adolescent is often sullen, withdrawn, and hostile. This is particularly so upon the first admission from an acute hospital. Prior to this moment, the youth had had fantasies of getting well and going home as did the other patients on the floor. But now he is faced with the chronicity and permanence of

* The ultimate sexual functioning of anyone disabled by a congenital or acquired cord lesion is a matter of intense, but often ignored, concern. According to Anderson and Cole, most afflicted females can participate in coitus and are fertile. Males face greater limitations. Somewhat more than half of a group of spinal-cord-injured men have reported that they were able to achieve penile erection and one-fourth could complete intercourse. But only 5 percent experienced orgasm and 3 percent ejaculation. These authors do suggest, however, that both sexes can achieve orgasm if there is some residual pelvic innervation, and sometimes even in its absence. They stress the importance of psychological factors and the ability of some patients to "reassign sensation from neurologically intact portions of the body to the genitalia and experience orgasm from that sensation in their fantasy."

The adolescent who is disabled will be as preoccupied with these matters, in pursuit of his sexual identity, as he is with matters of intellectual and vocational fulfillment. And he or she may well consider them most important of all, experiencing the greatest self-depreciation in this area. Yet the health care professional, the family, and the outside world all tend to avoid this matter and pretend the adolescent has no such concerns. Far from it. He or she has worries not only about future reproductive potential but also for present erotic feelings that are so ascendant during these years, for masturbatory interests, and for drives for heterosexual contact. A youth with rapidly progressive muscular dystrophy confessed to his doctor that he had had all of life's experiences and was ready to die with one exception. He yearned to know what intercourse was all about. Sympathetic parents and hospital staff located an equally sensitive and empathetic call girl who fulfilled the boy's needs one afternoon in the privacy of a single room on the ward. The youth was satisfied to have savored all that he thought life could bring him and was content.—A.D.H.

his problem, the probability of little if any return of function, and the fear of dependency. The adolescent becomes concerned about his educational, vocational, and sexual future, about life and death itself. Besides being depressed, he or she may also go into a period of mourning for lost functions.

Rejection, denial, or unwillingness to deal with the disability is also a frequent initial attitude of adolescents who have an acquired disability. They do not care to deal with the deficit or want to look at their problem. At the beginning they frequently and vigorously request to be left alone. This attitude is often associated with the unrealistic fantasy that "I will get better and be like I was." Such an example is the adolescent boy who lost both of his upper extremities in an accident. When first admitted for rehabilitation he was withdrawn. His participation in his therapeutic program was erratic and he preferred to be left alone in his room. At times he was also aggressive and subject to impulsive outbursts of anger during the early months. But through both individual and group sessions he was able to work out his depression, his guilt about the accident, and his denial of the disability to the point where he not only wore his prostheses but became proficient in their use and accepting of himself.

After the "initial shock" of being in a long-term hospital situation, there are mood fluctuations that are relatively predictable as rehabilitation progresses. With realization of the extent of the disability and some measure of acceptance, the adolescent usually becomes more actively involved in the program and mobilizes past strengths to bring to bear on the present situation. It is now that we see the different personality characteristics described before come into play. With increased functional capabilities, with or without appliances, and even in the absence of changes in physical or neurological status, the mood gradually becomes one of well-being. This is, however, significantly influenced by the parents' attitude toward the adolescent and also how he or she is accepted by other adolescents when home from the hospital on a weekend pass.

This optimistic mood persists until the prospect of being discharged becomes imminent. Fear then takes hold: "How will I manage at home? How will I get to school, if a school will accept me? I will be a burden on my parents who have had enough problems with me emotionally and financially already. Can't I stay a little longer?" Though the adolescent may have been involved in supportive therapy and these questions dealt with before, the realization that he or she will soon have to leave the protective environment of the hospital and consequent anxiety blocks out the memory of answers previously given. This will be so in spite of the fact that the adolescent may have gone home regularly for weekends. The teen-ager is not alone in these fears and doubts of his capabilities. His family are just as fearful.

What about the adolescent who has no family? This, too, can be a particularly difficult problem to resolve when discharge approaches. What had been available to the youth before when he was healthy may now be inadequate because of the disabiliy. This set of circumstances is particularly applicable to those youngsters who have been bounced around from one foster home to another or from one institution to another, for whom this is no longer a viable solution. Long used to disappointments and uncertainty, these teen-agers usually once again overtly express a fatalistic view about leaving the hospital with an attitude of "What will be will be." But under this façade of bravado there is anger, fear, and doubt as to what really lies ahead.

The adolescent who is disabled experiences all the same anxieties and concerns as do his healthy contemporaries. They must all deal with changing body image, changing family and peer relationships, and strivings for identity and independence. They confront their awakened sexuality and begin to form more intimate relationships; marriage becomes a real consideration. They must make decisions about educational and vocational goals that may well affect them for the rest of their lives. At the same time, they place great importance on their dress and appearance, on sports and school activities, on parties and dating. These normative concerns become all the more difficult for adolescents who are disabled. They may not be able to participate fully in the activities of their peers. They may experience rejection from a world not always accepting of those who are less than whole; or they may fantasize rejection where none exists, because of their own inadequate body image. They start to fear for their future, wondering if they can ever achieve the independence and fullness of life that all adolescents seek. Yet through understanding their special needs in dealing with their disability, together with firm emotional support, we can help these adolescents work within their handicaps to lead rewarding lives.

Adolescent fears can be expressed by the following quote from Sir Walter Raleigh: "Fain would I climb, but fear I would fall." An effective rehabilitation program will attempt to get the adolescent who is disabled to climb with pleasure and not fear falling.

chapter twelve

The Dying Adolescent

The prospect of death is the most difficult aspect of human existence for each of us to face. For the most part we ignore or deny our own mortality. But for members of the health care professions the nature of the services they render provides not only frequent reminders of their own personal vulnerability but also common confrontation with the tragic proof of professional fallibility and direct refutation of all they seek to accomplish. Physicians, nurses, and others closely involved will to some extent inevitably share feelings of helplessness, grief, loss, and even anger with the dying patient and his family.

Never is this more poignant than at the death of a child or adolescent, someone whose life has not yet been fulfilled in any substantial measure. It is all the more unacceptable as the increasing pace of technological and medical advances provides us with a growing armamentarium against disease and greater hope for prolonging life. This is particularly true in the United States and other developed nations characterized by emphasis on human values and individual rights, relatively high economic standards, and absence of frequent mass death phenomena such as famines, plagues, natural catastrophes, and annihilating wars. Each conception is regularly expected to result in the birth of a healthy infant who, in turn, is expected to live to a ripe old age. Any event to the contrary is viewed as unacceptable. We have little resignation to or acceptance of death.

DEATH AND DYING IN ADOLESCENCE

While much has been written about the meaning of death and its management, relatively little notice has been given to the adolescent. Yet there are some unique aspects for this age group. The adolescent's concept of death approximates that of an adult. With the arrival of abstract thought at the beginning of the second decade, the young person comes to perceive the reality, totality, and finality of dying. Yet it is also during the teen years when uncompromised idealism is at its peak and the search for values and ethics is often expressed in intense traditional and nontraditional religious beliefs. While fully comprehending the irreversible nature of physiologic death, it is common for adolescents also to invest it with some sort of spiritual continuation.

Even if the patient does believe in an afterlife, the impact of dying with all its deteriorating functions is particularly difficult for an adolescent to bear. Young people facing death are acutely aware of losing everything just at the point of achieving adult status and what they perceive to be its inherent perquisites of freedom of action and choice untainted by parental impositions. Many youths view their childhood years as a painful time to be endured until emancipation arrives and not with the idealized retrospective visions of a time of play, joy, and irresponsibility that adults often possess. The implicit loss of mastery and control and the diminution of autonomy that are consequences of serious disease also create their own set of problems, as does the deterioration of physical and sexual integrity because of the ravages of illness or mutilative chemical and surgical interventions. From so many aspects, dying teen-agers are the greatest mourners of their own fate.

A last point relates to the unique legal situation of the young person who is more than a child yet not quite adult and who is still subject to the decisions of his parents. Many youths, quite capable of forming their own opinions, are now doing so, even when they are contrary to parental wishes. The law is increasingly recognizing this fact; in some areas, including certain aspects of medical care, minors are gradually being endowed with rights of their own. The resulting conflict between the rights of adolescents and the rights of parents—which does not exist either for younger children or for those who have reached majority—bears significant implications for the management of teen-agers with potentially fatal illnesses. Should they be told their diagnoses? Should they be asked to consent to mutilative surgical procedures? Do they have full privilege of confidentiality in the patient-doctor relationships? Each of these questions must be answered individually, in light of the maturity of a given youth. But in most instances we would answer yes, for we believe that the dying adolescent has the inalienable right to be master of his life to the very end.

PARENTS AND THE DYING YOUTH

The impact of a young dying child upon his parents includes such matters as the termination of parental hopes for immortality through the life of their offspring, guilt over perceived causal responsibility, feelings of failure as their nurturing efforts no longer result in positive growth and development, and simple despair at the loss of a loved person (who also may be seen as an extension of themselves).

Additional problems arise when the child is an adolescent. All of the foregoing are equally operative but are further colored and confused by the processes of emancipation. A teen-ager who had begun to move away from home and to detach himself or herself from parents, often through variable degrees of alienating and confrontational behavior, may find it singularly distressing to be forced into a regressive, more dependent situation against all inner drives. In consequence, alienating and confrontational behavior may well be intensified toward the family. At the same time, the patient in fact needs his mother and father more than ever and must look to them to resume a more caring role. Parents of dying adolescents face special problems in understanding and meeting these conflicts.

THE HOSPITAL STAFF AND THE DYING PATIENT

The dying and death of a patient never fails to raise anxieties in the hospital staff. The genesis of these anxieties and the methods chosen to cope with them are multiple and often much more subtle and complex than first meets the eye. They depend upon the interplay between the emotional determinants of why the individual chose a health career, his or her ability to deal with the personal implication of death, and the ways in which any stress is commonly and customarily met, be this through withdrawal or action-oriented modes.

The physician, nurse, or others closely involved in patient care may have chosen his or her vocation because of the authority and power it bestows. Or it may have inherent dependency gratification wherein the professional is unconsciously seeking care for himself while caring for others. Further, the choice of medicine may have been determined, in part, through identification and as an expression of the "ideal self." Of particular significance to this chapter is the motivational factor of the professional's need to master and control his or her own fears of death and mortality through its prevention in others. This is not to imply that these issues are detrimental to professional functions but simply to point out some of the unconscious forces at play, for they are significant in understanding our own vulnerabilities in the face of death: can we mobilize mature helping modes or will we succumb to an inappropriate response? Young professionals face particular difficulties in caring for the dying youth. Not only are there all the painful implications of death itself, but the novice staff member, all too close in age to the terminally ill adolescent, is particularly subject to the process of countertransference and overidentification.

When faced with a dying patient and his family, the primary physician and nurse are looked to by all as strong, calm, and empathetic providers of unremitting hope and support. The patient and parents, who must literally place life in the hands of the hospital staff, further invest them with unrealistic powers, believing them capable of magical and heroic acts. But these professionals are as human as anyone else and are equally subject to object loss, frustration, guilt, and depression when faced by failure. This in turn manifests itself in a number of ways.

The most likely recourse is avoidance. Once little more can be medically done, the physician, in particular, may substantially limit his visits to the ward or bedside, coming only when absolutely necessary and for only brief periods of time. Avoidance may further be evidenced in preoccupation with the mechanics of care and physiologic dysfunction, ignoring the patient himself.

Avoidance may merge into and be reinforced by intellectualization, the major coping mechanism of the physician or nurse in dealing with professional stress. It allows for the effective handling of biological needs while keeping anxiety within manageable bounds. But the inevitable consequence of intellectualization is to place distance between staff and patient. Such detachment may well exacerbate feelings of isolation, personal devaluation, and despair in those who are terminally ill and deprive them of helpful emotional support.

The physician may also express his feelings of helplessness and guilt in frustrated anger, which only leads to further guilt. This vicious cycle may be compounded even more if patient and parents are experiencing similar feelings themselves and project their own rage onto the staff. An intolerable situation can result. Sensing the danger and destructiveness of this course, the physician may deal with it by further avoidance or, alternatively, by atoning through offering unreasonable and unproductive hope, by becoming overindulgent and overprotective, or by entering into a succession of increasingly heroic, but ultimately useless, procedures. Further, he may displace his anger onto other staff members instead of onto the patient and become irritable and difficult himself.

Last, all members of the health care team inevitably experience at least some degree of depression over the deteriorating course and final death of an adolescent whom they have known for any length of time. Little can be done to avert it. But it can be lessened and made tolerable simply by recognizing it with others, and using appropriate and happier interim diversions. The committed health care team cannot avoid mourning the coming death of a young person whom they have known well, nor fail to join the patient and parents in this process and its ultimate resolution.

THE COURSE OF A FATAL ILLNESS

Accidents, suicides, and malignancies are the most common causes of death in adolescence. In the first two instances demise may be immediate or may result in a terminal hospitalization of but a few hours or days. Neoplastic disease presents a different course with prolonged and cyclical periods of remission and exacerbation. While not so frequently encountered, we must also consider the end stages of other chronic diseases and, in particular, renal failure with the attendant problems of dialysis and transplantation.

Acute Death.   Death is more apt to be swift than lingering for those admitted in a terminal state consequent to an accident or suicide effort. These and similar situations, such as unexpected operative deaths or cerebral hemorrhage, are unheralded catastrophes. The family has little opportunity to prepare for loss. Parents experience an initial numbness and shock, followed by disbelief and denial, then an almost inconsolable guilt and despair. All these feelings virtually isolate parents from the support and comfort of the hospital staff. There is little the latter can do except to respect these responses and avoid thoughtless statements that may have implied recriminations, as when a physician defends his own failure by suggesting that earlier treatment or prompter recognition might have averted the present course. To the contrary, it is particularly important to attempt to reassure the family that everything was done that could have been done, in hopes of absolving them of unrealistic guilt.

Further, it is not wise to strive unduly for autopsy permission in this case. At these times parents are frequently close to the limits of endurance and also may have grossly distorted views of reality. The hospital staff are apt to be perceived as unwelcome strangers who have possibly even contributed to their child's demise. Pushing too hard for an autopsy under these circumstances will only result in further fixation of this understandable paranoid ideation and resistance, to the detriment of the family and the predictable failure of the attainment of staff goals. It also goes violently against the grain of human compassion.

Physicians and nurses are usually not directly emotionally involved in an acute death situation, tending to remain objective bystanders. Helpful professional assistance in the processes of the family's mourning and grief usually occurs after the period of hospitalization itself. The family's physician who knows them well plays a key role at this time.

However, a quite different state of affairs results when the initial physical assault leaves a living but comatose patient. The situation now takes on the characteristics of a chronic course. Additional problems accrue when vegetative life functions are being maintained indefinitely through external life support systems. These are often instituted after instances of serious head trauma or major surgery when the outcome is still in doubt. But once this commitment has been made, it often becomes virtually impossible to "pull the plug" unless the full "Harvard"-type criteria of death are met, (no evident brain wave function, etc.), even when it is obvious to all that any type of recovery is virtually impossible. The decision to use these ''heroic measures'' must be carefully weighed in advance of their application.

Chronic Deaths: The Stages of Dying.   The recognized stages of dying in the adult also pertain to the adolescent. According to Kübler-Ross, an initial denial of the diagnosis progresses to depression and anger, as the implications of the condition first become clear; then to bargaining, as either remission or some sort of equilibrium is temporarily achieved; and finally to resolution, as a type of premonitory mourning, when the inevitability of death is at last fully perceived. Although this sequence is unchanging, duration of the various stages may significantly differ from one individual to another. Or there may be fixation or retrograde movement at certain points, complicating matters still further.

These stages are often experienced by parents, paralleling those of their child. And hospital staff, often functioning *in loco parentis,* also tend to be vulnerable to some degree. Indeed, death and dying catch up all concerned in these inexorable processes.

MANAGEMENT

Goals.   Effective management of the dying adolescent seeks to achieve multiple goals. First, it is essential to gain the confidence and cooperation of the patient and his entire family. At the most simplistic level there are legal requirements of parental consent. In a more complex vein, conflicting views between a youth and his family or between staff and parents as to just what therapeutic course to pursue may activate a three-way struggle for control that can seriously impede care.

Second, it is important to encourage optimal function and provide for the adolescent's continued maturation as his illness permits. The youth must be enlisted as an active partner in care; dependency requirements and functional impairments must be minimized; and independence, mobility, and self-care must be promoted to the greatest degree possible. Normal adolescent activities, ongoing education, opportunities for social interaction with peers and others, and involvement in various compensatory activities are vital.

A particularly important point relates to pain. Adolescents, who tolerate discomfort poorly, often single out delays in medication or inadequate dosages as the greatest deficiency in their care. Effective and prompt analgesia *must* be given as needed throughout the course without the spurious, denying rationalization that the patient will become addicted. To deny the terminally ill adolescent as continuous a surcease from his pain as is possible because of a feared drug dependence is ridiculous.

The last of these goals is the development of a coherent and integrated philosophical approach. Based on a thorough knowledge of the family and an understanding of the psychological processes involved, this includes the maintenance of hope while it is still realistically justified and the provision of an adequate structure to help parent and patient deal with the terminal phase.

The Ward Structure.   Perhaps the cardinal rule in managing the dying patient is the promotion of helpful interstaff and staff-patient-family exchange. Failure to share and explore thoughts and emotions isolates each person from the other and leaves each to bear his or her own particular burden alone. This invariably leads to the promotion of inappropriate responses, blurred roles, and conflicting messages that result in additional anxiety and further maladaptation.

Optimal management depends upon a frank and open interstaff expression of feelings, the development of a closely coordinated team, clearly defined roles, and an assured transmission of information and plans among all concerned. To this end, regular "problem-solving" conferences are essential. Obviously, these should be attended by all involved professionals, including attending physicians, house staff, nursing staff, social service workers, recreational and occupational therapists, and teachers. Specialists, surgeons, and consultants should also be encouraged to join. The liaison psychiatrist and the consultant in adolescent medicine are indispensable.

In these conferences, staff feelings may be ventilated and to some degree understood. Problems in patient or parent management can be reviewed and remedial action planned. Medical or surgical therapeutics, prognostic expectations, or staff confusions over the patient's course are also matters to be taken up. The definitions of staff roles should address such matters as who will relay medical announcements and decisions to the family, who will prepare the youth for procedures and explain details, and who will offer opportunities for the patient or parents to talk. Plans should also be drawn up for meeting the youth's educational and recreational needs. It is important that all concerned present a united front and avoiding giving confused and conflicting messages to the patient, and that the totality of his needs be met.

The second key to effective management is the team approach. This depends upon open communication, both horizontally among members of different disciplines and vertically among the various levels of training and responsibility within each discipline. Verbal interchange is much more effective than chart notes, which always tend to be brief and relatively uninformative about all but the most basic medical matters. This also means that the patient's primary physician is responsible for regularly informing the staff of the direction and progress of care.

From the many staff members involved in a patient's care, he and his family tend to select one person in each discipline with whom they feel most comfortable and prefer to talk. These choices should be respected and fostered in the development of a *primary* ward care team. In general, this should consist of a mature nurse on each shift, a resident or fellow in adolescent medicine, and a social worker. New young nurses, interns, and medical students can and should provide supportive care. But usually they have not had sufficient experience to deal effectively with the dying patient and should not be asked to shoulder the primary burden. Announcements of new procedures, their consequences, or serious complications remain with the resident or fellow on his own or as agent of the private doctor, surgeon, or specialist involved. Reinforcement and ventilation becomes the major function of the nurse. Environmental support needs and unstable parents should get special attention from the social worker. The liaison psychiatrist enters in when inappropriate responses by the patient or parents seriously interfere with care or cause emotional distress that is impervious to the efforts of the team.

The ward attending physician, consultant in adolescent medicine, mental health consultant, and head nurse comprise the *secondary* or coordinating team. Their function is advisory to the staff on all patients through formal and informal meetings. Physicians at this level may also need to act as liaison between the primary care team and busy senior surgeons and specialists who have not generally been in close, prolonged contact with the patient and often enter the picture as but one of many involved in the management of a complex "case." Without such coordination the opportunities for breakdowns in relaying essential information and coordinating care are monumental. Indeed all the components of the weekly ward planning conference for regular patient care, as presented in chapter 7, are relevant here.

The Course. The vast majority of adolescents entering the hospital with suspected neoplasm (this condition is the model used because of its relatively greater incidence than other fatal diseases and its easy adaptability to other categories of serious chronic illness) have little idea as to the nature of their illness. Parents tend to be no better informed even though the family's physician may already have made a tentative diagnosis. There appears to be an unconscious effort on the part of all concerned to deny the potential for serious disease. It is not uncommon for the youth and his family to state that they are simply coming to the hospital for a few routine tests.

Usually there is also some degree of perception of the true state of affairs, as the symptoms of unexplained weight loss, unresolving masses, persistent bleeding, and other such dire manifestations are obvious in their significance. Consequently, one often finds much anxiety and ambivalence just below the surface denial and calm. The staff should not be surprised by ambiguous behavior during the first few days, and they should be prepared for a period of tension and confusion as diagnostic procedures are being carried out. Nurses and doctors can expect to be bombarded by the frequent inquiries of the patient and family about various test results, and at the same time may have to accept a relatively frustrating and passive role when parents protectively refuse to allow them to get too close.

This frequent questioning of virtually all known staff members who pass by the door can create awkwardness for the caring personnel who do not know how to respond, resorting instead to various equivocations and "buck passing." It may be far simpler just to avoid the patient. Regrettably, the family is thus isolated, and their protectiveness of the patient is further reinforced, until the "announcement" is made. The risk of alienation increases as time goes on and this conspiracy of silence is maintained.

It is far better that the family physician openly advise the parents at the very beginning that the condition could be serious. They are usually highly suspicious anyway. As matters are still conjectural, parents are able to cope reasonably effectively. Further, the primary physician—or specialist or surgeon if the patient has been referred—should have it clearly understood by the family that he will regularly report progress and that he alone is to be the provider of both good news and bad. Realistically, one cannot always depend on the specialist or surgeon fully to assume this role and, as previously noted, it should be shared by the physician member of the primary care team.

If, on receipt of a biopsy report, bone marrow findings, X-ray readings, or whatever, the diagnosis of malignancy is confirmed, the results must be conveyed to the parents. Frequently this creates a crisis. Parents tend to deny the diagnosis and often refuse to let the patient know what is happening. The physician often leaves without communicating either the content of his announcement or his therapeutic plans to the staff, who are left to deal with questions they feel ill equipped to handle. The distraught parents and the confused staff unconsciously communicate their feelings to the patient, creating new difficulties. Obviously, proper and timely use of the problem-solving conference can preclude this sorry state of affairs.

It is also important at this time for the staff to face and understand their own ambivalence, denial, and anxiety about death and dying. It is no crime to share grief with and for a patient and parents when one is close to them and the time is appropriate. On the other hand, one must maintain enough objectivity not to be pulled into the denial of reality or to act out inappropriately by deserting the patient and family when they most need support.

At this point it might be well to review the problem of what to tell the patient about his illness. Certainly the adolescent will by now have some awareness of its seriousness. Retrospectively, most youths with malignancies have advised us that they knew their diagnosis quite early in the course despite elaborate efforts to hide this knowledge from them. It is our contention that most adolescents are quite aware of their plight under any circumstances and that avoiding its open discussion deprives the youth of his rightful opportunity to work through his anxieties optimally, set his affairs in order, and prepare for a dignified death. On the other hand, we do not recommend immediate full revelation of all the facts. Rather, one can let the patient himself direct this matter, relatively assured that the youth will ask for no more information than he is able to manage at the given moment. Thus we feel that although no information should necessarily be hidden from a dying adolescent the timing and method of conveying it is of the essence.

First, as for parents, all information pertaining to the nature of the diagnosis, prognosis, and therapeutic plans should be given only by the primary caring physician. Second, this doctor should regularly spend time with the youth alone every day or two, establishing a climate of mutual trust and openness. Parents, roommates, visitors, and peripheral personnel should all be absent at this time. Occasionally it may be helpful to have the team staff nurse or social worker present to serve as advocate in assisting a youth who finds it difficult to ask questions about himself.

The patient should be encouraged to take the lead. This may be prompted by asking if he has any specific questions, worries, or concerns he would like to talk about. These inquiries should be backed by sound evidence of interest and immediate availability, such as sitting at the bedside. Asking perfunctory questions while standing in the doorway—obviously hoping for negative replies and eager to get on with other business—is both unresponsive and discouraging.

At first, seriously ill adolescents are most anxious about how their illness or therapy will interfere with their normal pursuits or affect their appearance. Most of their queries will address these points, denying the real implications of their disease. Until the youngster is better known and a good relationship established, it is best not to press matters too far, giving him only that information he is ready to hear. And while answers to the patient's questions should always be honest, one should also be sure of what he is really asking about. If the intent is uncertain or confused, it can be clarified by asking "Can you tell me a little more about what you have on your mind?" or something similar. If the true nature of the situation has not been fully revealed to the youth at the time of his first discharge, he should at least be told that he has a chronic or exacerbating disease and that he must cooperate with continued treatment and care.

Generally, there is little difficulty with any but the ultimate question: "Am I going to die?" The response to this is hard indeed. Probably the best answer is to point out to the patient that he has a very serious illness but that much can be done to make him feel better and to restore function and that he and the staff will work closely together toward these goals. We are committed to the view that adolescents should be advised of their diagnosis in terms they can well understand. But this should also be firmly coupled with all *realistic* prospects for cure or remission. If reasonable hope is a part of this discussion, one can assume that the young patient will—at least early in the course—quickly latch onto the most favorable aspects. He will experience less anxiety, be more cooperative, and in general cope with his situation more effectively once these matters have come out into the open. Nothing can be worse for the youth who knows he is seriously ill and who is sensitive to the distress and concern of those around him than to feel he is the victim of a conspiracy of silence and to be left alone in his fantasy to figure out what is going on.

By the time events have progressed to a more terminal stage, the youth all too well senses his impending death and usually ceases to ask questions on this count. If, however, the possibility of dying has not been discussed before, it may now come up for the first time. In response, one can only be honest, but with the firm statement that those staff members he is most comfortable with will be close by, throughout, doing all they can to make him comfortable and to help.

A most difficult problem arises when the patient asks about his diagnosis but his parents refuse to allow him to be told. This is a singular dilemma for the adolescent. Still a minor, he is legally and to some degree emotionally dependent on his parents and subject to their decisions made on his behalf. On the other hand, he is assuming ever greater responsibility for determining his own affairs and making his own decisions. The basic conflict rests in the rights of parents to control over their offspring and the right of the adolescent to be master of his own fate. To go against parental wishes has obvious implications both legally and for the maintenance of their trust and cooperation. But to refuse to respond to the youth with some degree of honesty may compromise the same qualities in the patient himself. The conflict is best resolved by convincing the parents that it is essential to help their child by allowing him to talk openly about his worries and fears.

To return to the management of the stages of dying. As the condition advances, the primary care team must focus on developing a strong supportive relationship with the patient, his parents, and his siblings in preparation for the time when depression, rage, and guilt will arise. These feelings may be manifested in both patient and parents in various ways: withdrawal, wrath, negativism, combative and complaining behavior, provocative acting out, or any other of the wide variety of responses to medical stress (see chapter 4). Food may become a special issue at this time, since the patient has usually become anorexic and parents may be panicky about his emaciated condition.

Often, such early signs of difficulty are missed or misunderstood. Regardless of the patient's or parents' behavior, however, it is critical that the staff accept the blast and tolerate variable degrees of ongoing negativism with understanding and sympathy. Because this is difficult to do, professionals tend to react with avoidance or counter-hostility. The problem-solving conference can be particularly useful to diffuse staff anger, helplessness, and depression. The primary physician best serves the patient if he visits often and assumes both a more authoritarian and a more rationalistic stance. This is accomplished by alternating between frequent, direct statements about the overall treatment plan itself on the one hand and more careful, empathetic explanations about necessary tests, procedures, therapies, and results on the other.

The focus of ward management is twofold. First is the maintenance of as much active, positive function on the part of the patient as is compatible with his medical status coupled with appropriate limits on his behavior. School, social, and recreational activities must continue as long as they can be physically tolerated. Allowing the abandonment of normal expectations and pursuits of the adolescent life style will only be interpreted by the patient as a negative message, deepening his despair and withdrawal. Further, it will reinforce feelings of resentment about his increased dependency needs and diminished mastery and control, insuring the loss of yet further self-esteem.

Second is the absolute prevention of isolation as a result of both passive withdrawal by the youth and active avoidance on the part of the staff. Desertion by physicians and nurses provides further signals of the hopelessness of the situation. It serves only to protract and intensify the patient's sense of despair and promotes feelings of rejection. In addition, the fantasies of adolescents and even the staff when faced with silence are usually much worse than when all are aware that a serious illness is present and they can talk about it openly. Additionally, while hope must always be held out, physicians must be careful in overdoing investigative and therapeutic procedures as a manifestation of their own denial, frustration, or guilt.

Management of the dying adolescent is a little like walking a tightrope and takes careful and continuous monitoring of the feelings of all concerned. But, if properly managed, the frequent guilt-engendered hostility and disagreement between one parent and the other begins to lessen; friction between patient, parents, and staff decreases; the family is able to spend a more realistic amount of time at home with siblings; and the youth is more calm and less anxious. These feelings of resolution are, of course, variable in duration, take place at different rates in different persons, and, like the disease itself, can move back and forth with remissions and exacerbations.

However, for certain parents or patients with premorbid emotional disability, resolution may not occur and there can be arrest at any point from the initial phase of denial on, coupled with a pathological degree of parental premonitory hovering. Such situations may require direct psychiatric intervention.

Most adolescents with a fatal illness experience a period of remission following the initial diagnosis and treatment. The cyclical course of exacerbation and remission can occur a number of times, although with each improvement the degree of restored function is usually substantially less than the time before. Nonetheless, each remission and the return of the patient to his home enhances hope and these times are relatively easier to bear and more emotionally tranquil, often allowing a reasonable amount of normal activity, pleasure, and diversion. These periods of remission are largely made difficult by parental overindulgence, excessive permissiveness, and overprotection. To be so differentiated from his siblings and from the parental attitudes that prevailed before he was ill can create its own particular problems for the adolescent and his family. It is far better if the youth can be treated normally as when he was well insofar as his stamina and medical requirements allow. The ward staff will need to help parents understand and accept this need before discharge.

Ultimately, these remissions give out and the last stage of terminal illness arrives. At first this may be responded to with an exacerbation of the earlier stages of denial, and reactivation of depression, negativism, and conflict. But shortly, through resolution, the youth then prepares for death. In our experience, it has been impressive to observe the degree to which adolescents protect their parents at the end of their lives. Close staff are often treated with a kindness and courtesy as well. It is a time of anticipatory grief and mourning and of bidding farewell to those who are loved. The pain of separation for all is real and is to be shared and openly communicated.

To stand or sit quietly by the adolescent's bedside, perhaps holding a hand, can offer more support and evidence of concern than any words. At this point, management—if it can be called that—consists of staying in close touch with the youth, demonstrating continued affection and caring and respect for his courage, assuring him he is not abandoned or alone and providing him with a peaceful, painless, and dignified death.

Staff need to be particularly careful not to succumb unrealistically to their own feelings of helplessness. This is not the time for heroic but pointless measures that merely stave off the inevitable, nor the time for unnecessary procedures and useless treatments that further subject the youth to pain, humiliation, and indignity. In this context there needs to be concise preplanning for the degree of life supports to be used.

For family members, the loss of their child is accompanied by a continuance of the process of mourning that to some extent began before the actual moment of death. Having an opportunity to review past events, to share a tear, and to think of the youth as he had once been is as necessary for involved physicians and nurses as it is for parents. Reassurance for all concerned that everything possible was done is also essential.

SPECIAL PROBLEMS

Care in the Teaching Hospital.   An inherent conflict between patient care and training prevails at most referral institutions. Yet many fatally ill adolescents find themselves in just such a setting. This is indeed an intricate problem, but teaching can continue without compromising care when the primary responsibility is not put in the hands of interns or other health care novices without very careful ongoing supervision. In general, the complexities of managing the dying patient and the anxieties particularly experienced by young staff suggest that the primary responsibility be borne by more experienced personnel rather than by those least able to handle feelings of anxiety, depression, and helplessness.

Treatment Controversies. Substantial controversy often exists over what therapeutic measures should be taken in a case. Considerations of effective treatment can run the gamut from euthanasia to nonintervention, from severe surgical mutilation to a conventional course of chemotherapy. The unfortunate results of such disagreements can be a plethora of mixed communications to patient and parents when the staff cannot resolve their ambivalence. Furthermore, there have been times when parents, in the face of overwhelming anxiety, have had to make one of a number of important choices they ill understood because of the physician's indecision. Obviously such conflicts need to be worked out, a consensus reached, and a unified approach presented.

This may be particularly difficult when various staff members do not agree with the course instituted by the senior physician. But his views need to be respected and, while he may be engaged in honest but private argument, his final decision must be supported and his authority in the eyes of the patient and parents not undermined.

Dying at Home. When death is inevitable and there are no further available therapeutic measures, the decision of whether the youth should die at home or in hospital may arise. While in this country it seems generally expected that dying should take place in the hospital, there are valid arguments for its occurrence at home where the youth may be peacefully surrounded by those he cares for in his natural environment. Here he also will not be distressed by the noise, comings and goings, unfamiliar people, and assorted treatments of the hospital setting.

There is much to commend this approach, but careful assessment of the situation is indicated before it is taken. Are the parents able to cope with both their own and the patient's emotions and his nursing needs or do they need the continued support and help of the staff they have come to know and trust over past admissions? What would be the impact of this course upon the other children? Their exposure to the moment of death of a family member may be an unacceptably upsetting experience. Negative evaluations on either of these counts will mitigate against the advisability of the youth's dying at home. But optimistic prospects for this alternative may provide the opportunity for a closeness and special meaning to the moment of death that only being at home affords. If the patient is in a referral institution some distance away, a good compromise can be made by the transfer to a local hospital.

Dialysis and the Patient's Choice to Die.   A particularly difficult problem is that of the adolescent on dialysis while awaiting a transplant. It is difficult indeed for an adolescent to handle the rigors and dependency requirements of dialysis and the profound oral deprivations of the concomitant dietary restrictions for more than a few months. Even with psychiatric help, school and peer group functions become virtually paralyzed and emotional well-being seriously compromised. Depression over these events coupled with the potentiating effects of feeling chronically unwell can often serve to frustrate even the most well-worked-out program for psychological support until a transplant can be accomplished.

When no kidney is forthcoming over a prolonged period of time or when transplantation has repeatedly failed it may be the active choice of the patient to terminate dialysis and die. When these wishes have been consistent over a period of time and he or she no longer consents to this treatment, when no hope of a life free of these supports exists and when parents concur, it must be viewed as the patient's right to choose death instead, as difficult as this may be to accept.

CONCLUSION

The management of the dying adolescent can be both the most difficult, exhausting, and emotionally painful experience and yet, at the same time, the most gratifying and important of the tasks that a hospital staff can be called upon to undertake. One needs all one's personal resources to face the helplessness and anxiety that our upbringing and culture have imposed on our attitudes toward death—especially in the young. Only when these attitudes are faced, shared, and modified can the real work of helping patient and family take place.

chapter thirteen
Consent and Confidentiality

Many health care professionals tend to assume that parental consent is an absolute prerequisite to the treatment of all minors except in the most dire of emergencies. This is simply not true. Traditional legal determinants have always permitted a variety of exceptions, and are now rapidly giving way to new concepts as well. Thus there is much more flexibility today than is generally recognized.

The aforementioned "traditional" view basically stems from old common law pertaining to both contracts and torts. This has been widely interpreted to hold that medical care constitutes a contractual relationship between the patient and physician. As a minor is not deemed competent to enter into any contract on his own, this could only be validly carried out by the parent or legal guardian on the minor's behalf. If a doctor were to touch a minor without such a valid contract (consent), this would constitute an unauthorized touching, or assault and battery. But, when such matters do come to litigation, this is nearly always heard in civil rather than criminal courts, since no intent to harm is involved.

It has been this set of deductions, based on a body of general provisions rather than specific defining statutes, that has led to the widespread belief that parental consent is an immutable component of a minor's health care. In fact, it has only been since 1973 that parental consent has been definitively mandated in a number of states and this only in relation to abortions. But, as we shall later point out, these same statutes have just recently been largely struck down as unconstitutional by the Supreme Court.

WHAT IS "THE LAW"?

It is important to our further discussions to keep in mind that "the law" is comprised of a number of factors, all of which can be called upon in defense or prosecution of a case. The ultimate decision as to whether a given action was in fact legal is for the courts on weighing the merits of the argument of each side.

Statutes are the expressions of legislative intent, directive in and of themselves. But frequently these laws are very general, ambiguous, or unclear, and subject to different interpretations—or they may be specific but fail to cover a new situation. For example, one may be most uncertain about just how broadly to interpret provisions relating to the emergency treatment of minors without parental consent when what constitutes an "emergency" is not defined. In another instance, there are a number of relatively recent laws that allow minors to consent to services related to "the treatment and prevention of pregnancy." There are few clues here as to whether this phrasing should or should not be held to include the performance of abortion as well (this is, after all, a form of treatment of pregnancy).

Because of such confusions, both state and federal court decisions also comprise a very significant part of "the law," especially when these are interpreting unclear statutes or deducing the appropriate rule to cover a new problem. Later, we shall discuss in detail those decisions contributing to the emerging "mature minor doctrine" in relation to medical care.

A statute may be quite clear in its intent, but unconstitutional nevertheless. Thus, when a state seeks to impose a given set of conditions or standards by legislation, the courts may find that this either unjustifiably deprives the individual of his rights or is unwarrantedly discriminatory and invalidate it. A case in point is the United States Supreme Court decision in *Brown* v. *Board of Education* (347 U.S. 483, 1954) prohibiting racial segregation in schools and upholding the right of all children to an equal education.

Then there is "the law in fact." Insofar as we can determine, there has never been an instance in which a physician was held liable for damages in treating a minor over the age of 15 years on his own consent for any matter, nor for providing contraceptive services to a minor of any age. "The law in fact" can also be found in the interpretive guidelines of official agencies or recognized institutions. Thus, despite the absence of specific enabling statutes, the New York State Department of Social Services, acting on DHEW family planning guidelines, now requires that all sexually active minor welfare recipients must be given the opportunity to receive contraceptive services regardless of age. And New York City municipal hospitals have provided such services to any minor requesting them on her own consent for several years. Many private hospitals and physicians have based their own standards of practice on these guidelines as well. And, to our knowledge, these policies have yet to be challenged in the New York courts.

Federal and local strictures relative to monetary appropriations may also be relevant. To illustrate, under the Family Educational Rights and Privacy Act of

1974, schools are now subject to the curtailment of all federal funding that they receive if parents are in any way denied the opportunity to review all their child's educational records on request. Thus, while the withholding of these records from parental review is not a specifically prohibited act in and of itself, the penalties that may result from failing to comply with these regulations are indeed compelling.

Last, common and customary practice also has a bearing on determining what "the law" is. Virtually all "free clinics," adolescent medical clinics, and family planning centers in the country now treat a significant number of minors on their own consent when their health requires it, even in the absence of specific authorization under state law. Moreover, it is widely held by experts in the field that the preservation of confidentiality in the doctor-patient relationship is critical to the effective rendering of adolescent health care.

Thus "the law" can be seen as a complex interplay between a variety of factors and is comprised of existing statutes; their variable interpretation under case law—either in terms of what the courts hold to be their legislative intent or in relation to their constitutionality; local and federal guidelines; policies of official agencies or recognized organizations; and common and customary practice. All may be looked at to infuse meaning into archaic and often vague legal restrictions.

"PARTIAL EMANCIPATIONS"

Another set of factors that supports our position that parental consent requirements are hardly absolute, relates to what might be termed "partial emancipations." Thus minors have always been permitted to function as adults in certain selected areas. A young person may drive a car substantially in advance of his majority; may be a bootblack, baby sitter, or paper boy even before his teens; can seek wider employment upon reaching the age of 14; is no longer subject to compulsory school attendance after his sixteenth year; may be tried in adult criminal courts at this same age; or may, if female, consent to sexual intercourse variably between 12 and 18 years (depending on the particular state) in that she is no longer subject to statutory rape laws. Well before the present widespread lowering of the age of majority from 21 to 18 years, minors of this lesser age had still further adult prerogatives: all limitations on employment became lifted; many females and some males could consent to marriage; and young men could be asked to defend their country by the draft. This list is by no means complete, but it more than serves to demonstrate the significant degree to which the law has long bestowed adult privileges and responsibilities upon minors well in advance of their majority. Legislatures clearly have never intended for the minority status to be without exception, particularly when it concerns matters of "person" (in contrast to "property"). And the graduating ability of adolescents to function in a responsible way, paralleling their developing maturity, is firmly taken into account.

MINORS' RIGHTS

A brief digression into this realm will further demonstrate the growing recognition of the minor as an individual in and of himself, clearly entitled to constitutional guarantees. Prior to the mid-1960s, the courts had rarely viewed children and minor adolescents as having rights of their own as did adults. Instead they were almost wholly subject to the will of parents, guardians, and social institutions, and to the decisions that these parties made on their behalf. A vast array of protective laws were enacted in the "best interests" of the child. This included such matters as prohibitions against abuse and neglect; compulsory school attendance; restrictions on employment; child welfare laws; and the establishment of the juvenile justice system.

But, beginning in 1964, a significant change began to take place. The first intimations occurred with the United States Supreme Court's decision *In re Gault* (387 U.S. 1, 1967). Gerald Gault, age 15, had had the poor judgment to make an obscene telephone call to one of his less favored teachers. In turn she filed charges against him. The Arizona Juvenile Court ultimately remanded the boy to a state farm for an indeterminate term, but which could be as long as six years, or until his twenty-first birthday. Gerald, like so many other youths subjected to juvenile court proceedings, had been denied virtually all of the protections mandatory for adults under the Bill of Rights. Among other omissions, his accuser had never testified or even appeared in court; Gerald was not given the right to cross-examine or informed of his right against self-incrimination; and his right to counsel was curtailed. Further, he was not notified of the charges levied against him until the day of the hearing, and he was not given a transcript of the proceedings for purposes of appeal.

In this and several subsequent cases, the Supreme Court has come to accord minors almost all of the provisions of the Bill of Rights. However, it has not yet gone so far as to extend them the right to bail or trial by jury. While acknowledging the many deficiencies of present-day juvenile justice, the Court continues to hold that minors should not be deprived of the ideal and protective prospect of closed, secret, and rehabilitative proceedings, and that they will be less benefited by the open and adversarial nature of a jury trial.

In a slightly later and even more far-reaching case (*Tinker* v. *The Des Moines Independent School District,* 393 U.S. 503, 1969), the Supreme Court ruled that minors could no more be deprived of their freedom of speech than could adults. In this instance, three young teen-agers had joined their parents in protesting the Vietnam War by wearing black armbands. The principal of their school responded by declaring that anyone wearing such a band in class would be suspended. The youngsters continued their protest and were forced to leave school. The Supreme Court, in reversing the lower court's decision in favor of the school authorities, once and for all established that the right to freedom of speech was for all citizens and could not be curtailed on account of age or student status.

It is, however, significant that in each of these instances the young plaintiffs had full parental support in pursuing their cases, and the true adversary was always external to the family unit. The problem posed by a dispute that clearly divides the minor and his parents was not in contest. Nor was this at issue in other important Supreme Court decisions pertaining to minors such as *Brown* v. *Board of Education* in ruling against discrimination in education, or *Goss* v. *Lopez* (43 U.S. Law Week 4181, Jan. 21, 1975), which held that high school students facing temporary suspension from a public school are entitled to notice and hearing and that this cannot be arbitrarily imposed. Moreover, the Court seems specifically to have avoided this matter in its 1973 landmark decision on abortions (*Roe* v. *Wade,* 410 U.S. 113, 1973; *Doe* v. *Bolton,* 410 U.S. 179, 1973). While it has been firmly established that there is a constitutional right to privacy and that this obtains to the doctor-patient relationship for adults (*Griswold* v. *Connecticut,* 381 U.S. 479, 1965; *Eisenstadt* v. *Baird,* 405 U.S. 438, 1972), it has yet to be determined to what extent this right devolves on minors (see footnote, page 232).

But trends in lower court decisions do give direction here, and exceptions to the absolute powers of parents in consenting to the health care of their minor child abound. Health care professionals will be quite familiar with the option of asking the courts to assume temporary guardianship when parents refuse to allow life-saving blood transfusions out of religious principles. Nor is parental consent in question when reporting a child suspected of being abused. But these are instances where the state takes over for parents in what it views to be in the best interests of the child, without consideration of what a minor might view as his own best course.

But this too is changing. We have noted that a number of states have recently attempted to control a minor's access to abortion by statutorily requiring parental consent for this procedure in individuals under the age of 18. But these laws have now been ruled unconstitutional in a number of instances (Florida, Kentucky, Colorado, Washington, Utah, Massachusetts, the District of Columbia, Pennsylvania, and Indiana). Only in Missouri has such a law been upheld, and even here implementation has been stayed by the U.S. Supreme Court pending appeal.

The April 1975 decision of a three-judge federal court in Massachusetts is illustrative of this new direction (*Baird et al.* v. *Bellotti,* Civil Action 74-4992-F, D.C. Mass., 1975). While the court acknowledged that parents do have rights and obligations in acting on behalf of their minor offspring, it further held that the requiring of parental consent for a minor's abortion set up rights for parents that were potentially at conflict with the interests of the girl. The court said:

> It is not they [the parents] who have to bear the child. Once born, the minor, and not they, will be responsible for it in all senses, financially and otherwise. It is difficult to think of any self-interest that a parent would have that compares with those significant interests of the pregnant minor.

The decision went on to point out that there is no "factual magic" in setting 18 as the age when a minor is mature enough to give an informed consent for abortion, and "that a substantial number of females under the age of 18 are capable of forming a valid consent." The U.S. Supreme Court heard this and the Missouri decisions in its 1975–76 terms. Their ruling, when handed down, will undoubtedly have significant implications for all aspects of a minor's health care.

In closely related decisions, the Maryland Supreme Court ruled that a parent could not force an unmarried pregnant minor to have an abortion against her will (*In re Smith,* 16, Md. App. 209, 195A. 2nd 238, 1972). And the Superior Court of the District of Columbia affirmed the reverse in stating that a parent could not prevent a pregnant minor from having an abortion if the minor desired it (*In re P.J.,* 12 Crim. L. Report 2549, D.C. Sup. Ct., Feb. 6, 1973). The growing trend is clearly in support of minors' rights to privacy and to determine their own biological fate, at least insofar as pregnancy and abortion are concerned.

THE "MATURE MINOR DOCTRINE"

The preceding decisions also lend firm support, if not outright direction, to the broader issue of the rights of minors in all health care matters. And, when taken together with yet other court decisions, constitute what is coming to be collectively called the "mature minor doctrine" or "mature minor rule." This principle holds that minor individuals who have achieved sufficient maturity as to be able to understand the risks and benefits of the treatment they are to receive are indeed capable of giving a valid informed consent. Thus, as previously noted, we can discover no instance in which a physician was found liable for treating a minor over the age of 15 years on his consent alone for any matter including surgery.

An example is the case of *Bach* v. *Long Island Hospital* (49 Misc. 2d 201, 267 N.Y.S. 2d 289, Supreme Court, Nassau County, 1966) in which a 19-year-old girl had agreed to a biopsy for a skin condition without parental consent.

(Note that this was well before minors came to be widely accorded majority at age 18 rather than 21.) In ruling on subsequent assault charges filed by the girl against her surgeon, the court held:

> In this case there is nothing to suggest that the plaintiff at the time of executing consent had not reached the age of discretion, or that plaintiff was under any physical or mental disability. Plaintiff's consent to the surgical procedure involved was a personal right which was validly exercised.

As long ago as 1935, in *Sullivan* v. *Montgomery* (155 Misc. 448, 279 N.Y. Supp. 575, City Ct. of N.Y., Bronx Cty., 1935), it was ruled that a 20-year-old youth could consent to anesthesia and the setting of his fractured ankle. In *Gulf & S.I.R. Co.* v. *Sullivan* (119 So. 502, Sup. Ct. Miss., 1928) a parental claim against the defendant for allowing their 17-year-old son to consent to a vaccination against their objections was disallowed on the grounds that the boy was sufficiently intelligent as to be able to understand the treatment and its consequences. And in *Lacey* v. *Laird* (139 N.E. 2d 25, Sup. Ct., 1956) where an 18-year-old girl had consented to plastic surgery on her nose and subsequently brought an assault charge against her surgeon, the court said:

> A charge that the 18-year-old plaintiff could not consent to . . . a simple operation would seem inconsistent with the conclusion of our General Assembly that any female child of 16 can prevent taking of liberties with her person from rape merely by consenting thereto at the time such liberties are taken. . . . The performance of a surgical procedure upon an 18-year-old girl with her consent will ordinarily not amount to assault and battery for which damages may be recoverable even though the consent of the girl's parents or guardian has not been secured.

EMANCIPATION

Definitions of emancipation, or those circumstances under which a minor will be exempted from the ordinary limitations of these years, are also expanding. For some time, even without enabling statutes, this status has widely been accorded married minors, those who are in the armed forces, or those who are living away from home with parental concurrence and self-supporting via bonafide employment. But a broader view frequently obtains, and minors who are still living at home but earning more than half their own support will also usually find themselves emancipated; as may those who have graduated from high school, or those who are parents themselves. Some alienated minors who have left home may also be able to defend their emancipation solely on the grounds that they are managing their own financial affairs and making all major decisions about the conduct of their lives, and this without regard to the degree of parental concurrence or the source of income. (However, it will still be difficult for most adolescents who live away from home under ambiguous circumstances to gain widespread adult acceptance of their self-declared independence.) These new concepts of emancipation provide a further expansion in the number of minors who are eligible to consent to their own health care.

MINOR'S-CONSENT-TO-HEALTH-CARE STATUTES

The Problem.   Despite the previous arguments, most physicians and hospitals remain unconvinced as to their quite strong legal position in treating mature or emancipated minors on their own consent. Even when they are convinced, criteria for defining emancipation and maturity in relation to consenting to health care are usually vague and imprecise. Moreover, few professionals wish to face the tribulations of a court action, even if they are sure to win. Most understandably, they look for strong guarantees of immunity from ever being prosecuted at all. The present malpractice threat is great enough as it is without adding the further risk of an assault and battery charge.

The Need.   There is no basic dispute with the position that many parents can be highly supportive to their adolescent offspring, and teen-agers certainly benefit from all the help they can get in the processes of growing up. Nonetheless, minors are often in pragmatic need of being able to obtain confidential health care on their own consent. This situation is most apt to occur in relation to venereal disease, pregnancy (prevention, diagnosis, and treatment), drug or alcohol abuse, some psychiatric difficulties, and other similar private matters that teen-agers may feel they simply cannot speak to their parents about and do not wish them to know. When minors afflicted in these ways believe parental consent will be required for treatment or that their confidences will be readily passed on, the inevitable consequences are to put off seeking help at all, or delay it to the point of serious detriment.

These same arguments also apply to alienated or runaway adolescents. Here the problem is not so much the particular nature of the need, but the existence of so much intrafamily conflict that communications have broken down and the minor rejects any parental involvement at all. Moreover, it is precisely in those homes with the greatest amount of discord wherein teen-agers are the most likely to act out in ways that will place their health in jeopardy. Thus, alienated adolescents are doubly in need of being able to consent to their own health care.

Apart from these pragmatic aspects, the pure and simple right of minors to consent to their own medical treatment and determine the fate of their bodies is also at issue. There is much to support the contention that when an adolescent is sufficiently mature as to able to understand the nature of the treatment he or she is to receive, this alone is sufficient to establish eligibility in the manner of self-consent.

Solutions.   A wide variety of state laws have now been enacted addressing these points. In essence, they all provide "partial emancipation" for the purpose of obtaining health care, but the precise qualifications for eligibility are highly variable from state to state. In the majority of statutes, a number of concrete factors are determining. This includes such matters as the patient's age (minors have been enabled to consent to all health care anywhere from 14 to 19 years); life style (that is, married, a parent, a member of the armed services, a high school graduate, not living at home and managing his or her own financial affairs); the particular medical problem at hand and services to be rendered (that is, limiting eligibility only for services related to venereal disease, pregnancy, contraception, or drug abuse, and so on); or some combination of these factors comprising a sort of "omnibus" law.

In an effort to be still more flexible, an increasing number of states (Mississippi, Kansas, Michigan, Arkansas, New Hampshire, and Ohio) have developed laws incorporating the broad principles of the mature minor doctrine. These statutes generally stipulate that a minor may consent to all his own health services if he or she is of "sufficient intelligence (or maturity) as to be able to understand the nature and consequences of the services they are consenting to." The obvious problem here is that it is difficult to come up with a yardstick by which one can measure "intelligence," "maturity," and "understanding."

It is virtually impossible to give all combinations and permutations here. For not only are each state's laws tremendously varied one from the other, but within each jurisdiction itself there is continuing change and evolution. Not only is this a "hot" issue (that is, parental rights over their minor child), but it is also in the vanguard of expanding minors' rights in a constitutional sense. Further, as noted earlier, determinants of just when a minor can consent to treatment on his depends on a number of other matters as well as statutory law. Specific information on these matters for any given state can often be obtained from that state's attorney general. Local departments of health and hospitals and regional Planned Parenthood offices are also generally well up on minor's consent laws in their locale. Additional valuable information can be found in the *Family Planning/Population Reporter* in relation to the latest in case and in statutory law. Other citations given in our bibliography are also helpful.

But some general trends do exist. Statutes in a majority of states generally allow persons who have reached their eighteenth birthday, or who are or have been married, or who are parents, or are in the armed services to consent to all aspects of their own health care. And traditionally emancipated minors have always been deemed eligible even if not legislatively spelled out (that is, those who are living away from home with parental permission, working in bonafide employment, and supporting themselves).

Every state, bar none, now has laws enabling minors to receive services related to venereal disease without parental consent. The last holdout, Wisconsin, finally gave way in 1975. While eleven states impose minimum age restrictions of anywhere from 12 to 14 years, minors of all ages are eligible in the rest.

There is a somewhat less widespread acceptance of pregnancy-related services. But twenty-eight states clearly provide for pregnancy detection and routine prenatal care on the minor's own consent, and usually without regard to age as well. Some twenty states have similarly eased restrictions on obtaining contraception. And in a handful abortion is also clearly within the province of a minor's consent. But, as noted before, yet other states have specifically prohibited this step. Whether such denying provisions will all hold constitutional water, so to speak, will be shortly determined by the U.S. Supreme Court. Advance conjectures suggest they will not and ultimately will be struck down.

Only a few states have specifically addressed the issue of drug and alcohol abuse or psychiatric care. Perhaps this is because advocates for legal change relative to minors' consent have been less vigorous in these areas than they have in expanding minors' rights in general or in addressing the urgencies of sex-related health care.

EMERGENCY CARE

Another evolving area relative to parental consent requirements will be found in the redefinition of what constitutes an emergency. Although there has never been any real question about the defensibility of rendering care in the absence of parents when the minor's life is at stake, this is not quite so well defined when the situation is still urgent but bodes something less than imminent demise. In addition, there may be considerable question as to whether the relief of pain or emotional distress is to be considered an emergency service as well. Many hospitals and physicians take a strict view of this matter, with frequent long delays in instituting care for children and adolescents while attempts to locate parents are made. A prompt, humane, and compassionate response to minors in pain and distress is often set aside in favor of avoiding any legal risk. Moreover, the possible longer-range complications of failing to render needed care (when life is not in question) must be taken into consideration.

CASE 69.   A 15-year-old male sustained a facial laceration in a school accident. A piece of glassware had exploded in the chemistry laboratory and a fragment of glass had become deeply imbedded in the boy's cheek. Surgery (and anesthesia) would be required to remove it. His parents were out of town overnight and neither they nor other relatives could be reached. The boy had been left on his own for the brief time that they would be away. As life was not in danger, it was decided that the legally prudent step would be to defer any treatment until the parents returned. The boy was simply placed in a holding unit overnight. But, by the following day, when the parents had arrived on the scene and their consent was obtained, there were evidences of infection and it was now felt unwise to suture the wound. The glass fragment was removed, antibiotics were administered, and the cut was allowed to heal on its own. The resultant disfiguring scar ultimately had to be surgically revised.

CASE 70.   A 13-year-old girl came to the emergency room by herself for treatment of fever and sore throat. Her husbandless mother both worked and took care of four younger children and could neither afford to give up even part of a day's pay nor to hire a baby sitter in order to accompany the patient (who was not really very ill). Because the girl was febrile, the hospital deemed it permissible to examine her. And this revealed tonsillitis, presumably due to beta hemolytic streptococcus. But because she was in no immediate danger it was decided that parental consent was necessary for the administration of a penicillin injection. As the family did not have a phone, the girl was given a consent form for her mother to sign and have notarized, together with the instructions to return with this the next day. The girl did not show up and was not seen again until several weeks later when she was admitted with acute glomerulonephritis, a direct complication of her original untreated illness. It turned out that the girl had become much better the day after the emergency room visit. Further, the mother did not know what a notary was, much less where to find one or pay for his services. So, all in all, it had not only seemed unnecessary to come back, but much easier to follow this course.

CASE 71.   A 14-year-old girl appeared in the emergency room alone. She asked to see a doctor but would not say why. As she did not appear ill, had no fever, and would not state her complaint, it was felt that no emergency existed and that she could not receive care without parental consent. She was so advised and sent home. The girl reappeared a month later in a very agitated state. On this count it was decided that a physician should at least talk to her. In the privacy of this contact, the girl stated that she was pregnant and requested an abortion. Once again she was told that her parent would have to accompany her for any treatment to be given at all. However, this time an appointment was made for both to see a social worker. But the girl was no more able to advise her family at this time than she had been before and let matters slide once again. Yet another month passed before desperation forced her to tell her mother. The pair quickly came to the hospital and parental consent for the abortion was at last obtained. But so much time had now passed that the pregnancy was too advanced, and an abortion could not be done.

A number of states are now responding to these and similar dilemmas by seeking ways of redefining the scope of emergency care in somewhat broader terms. In New York "medical, surgical, dental, health, and hospital services" may be rendered minors in the absence of parental consent when attempting to contact parents would result in such a delay in care as to "increase the risk to the patient's life or *health.*" A recent Massachusetts law stipulates that an emergency exists when the failure to institute prompt treatment would endanger "life, limb, or *mental well being.*" Delaware deals with this problem in somewhat more categorical form by permitting emergency services to be provided without parental consent for "any laceration, fracture or other traumatic injury," for "communicable disease," or for "any exposure to toxic substances. . . . which if untreated may reasonably be expected to threaten life or health." But in all these instances the decision as to what indeed constitutes a threat to "life or health" is left up to the treating physician to decide. Many doctors find such a responsibility disquieting and continue to take a narrow view. But, in light of the extremely expansive interpretation that has generally been given to the word *health* in other matters, there is every reason to believe that legislatures intend for these new emergency statutes to be considerably more inclusive than they have been in the past.

Other states have met this problem by providing for another adult to act *in loco parentis* when the patient's own parents cannot be reached. This could be a relative, school authority, or other person responsible for the child at the time the illness or injury occurs. This approach sidesteps attempting to define what an emergency is, while still allowing for both the institution of prompt treatment and the protective concern of an outside adult.

All in all, concepts of an emergency are expanding to include significant risk to physical and emotional health as well as simply to life. And there is increasing agreement that minors should not be required to endure unnecessary pain or be subject to the possibility of a less desirable course because of the inability to obtain parental consent. Further support for treating adolescents in emergency situations is also forthcoming from the mature minor rule.

One might well argue that physicians and hospitals could be even more liable for charges of negligence in failing to treat a condition as an emergency or under the mature minor rule when complications do ensue, than they would be for assault and battery in the course of clearly benefiting the child. The previous case histories are all to the point; in each instance the patient was both in urgent need of care and quite capable of giving an informed consent for the treatment involved. It is not inconceivable that negligence suits could be successfully brought against the treating physician and hospital on behalf of such youths, charging that they were denied the right to consent and that in consequence they had suffered unnecessary physical and emotional harm.

IMPLICATIONS FOR HOSPITALIZED YOUTHS

The issue of a minor's ability to consent and need for confidentiality are certainly more commonly encountered in ambulatory care, and less so on the ward. For few adolescents enter the hospital without the full knowledge and concurrence of their parents. But these matters do arise sufficiently often, both on the ward itself and in consideration of admission from the emergency room, as to make this important here as well.

In some instances the admission itself will be occasioned by highly sensitive and private matters such as second trimester abortions, delivery of a term pregnancy, drug detoxication or overdose, medical complications of substance abuse, and the like. It is not unusual at all for a minor in these circumstances to wish his condition to remain his own private affair. In other circumstances, intimate health problems and special confidences may well be uncovered in a youth admitted for some other need.

CASE 72. A 15-year-old girl was admitted for hepatitis some six weeks after her best friend had had the same disease. Although she was not considered in serious risk at all, she felt poorly and there was no one home in the day to take care of her. Her parents were divorced and her mother worked. Routine medical history unexpectedly revealed that the girl had missed her last menstrual period and believed herself to be pregnant. The existence of a first trimester gestation was confirmed. She very much wanted an abortion, and preferably before she went home. But she was adamant that her mother not know. Her parents' difficulties had culminated in bitter arguments over an older stepsister who had also become pregnant out of wedlock and had ultimately been banished from the home. The patient, with good reason, feared the same consequences for herself.

But, despite the extenuating circumstances, the hospital's counsel still felt that her wishes could not be met, although her confidences could be respected and her mother not told. A sympathetic aunt was advised of the problem and agreed to help, arranging for the abortion to take place in a local clinic as soon as the girl was discharged. This course was successfully pursued.

A third situation may be encountered among alienated minors who, while not clearly emancipated in traditional terms, have either left home or still reside with their families, but without any real communication. Here it is not so much the nature of the condition that prompts the minor's desire to keep his admission from his parents as much as it is that he does not wish to be reunited with them on any terms.

CASE 73. A 17-year-old male appeared in the emergency room complaining of abdominal pain and dark, tarry stools. He knew he had had an ulcer the year before and believed it to be acting up again. He was found to be moderately anemic and appeared to have lost some blood. Admission was indicated. But his life was not in immediate danger, nor was he in any acute distress. The patient requested that hospitalization be on his own consent and his parents not told. For he had long been having difficulty at home with an abusive and alcoholic father and passive mother who sided with her husband in all matters. The boy had finally left home several weeks before and was living with a friend. His parents did not know where he was and the youth wished it to remain that way.

The emergency room physician felt that not only was the boy quite mature enough as to be able to give an informed consent, but that he also had many qualifications of being an emancipated minor under newer definitions. Moreover, the situation itself could certainly be considered as an emergency in light of the possibility for a serious hemorrhage. Despite all these points and the hospital's own written policies supporting these moves, the administrative duty officer was still not entirely convinced. It was late at night and counsel could not be reached. He conceded that the youth could indeed consent to care, given all these circumstances, and allowed him to be admitted—but not without some misgivings. Just to be on the safe side, the administrator called and advised the boy's parents of what had been done anyway!

When the question of self-consent and confidentiality occurs in the course of admission, the patient is certainly at least entitled to a full assessment of the facts and a carefully rendered decision on whether he is eligible or not. Contributing to this decision will be existing enabling state statutes; the applicability of the mature minor rule; the minor's status vis-à-vis emancipation; whether or not an emergency exists in its various possible definitions; whether parental involvement will truly benefit the minor and whether the latter can be convinced of this fact; and the existence of intrafamily difficulties that might make it actually detrimental for the patient if parents were to know.

Whether a physician or hospital would or would not be found liable by the courts for breach of contract in treating a minor on his own consent and then notifying his parents against his will has yet to be tested. But in all probability such would not occur. The vast preponderance of minors' consent statutes are primarily enabling rather than compelling. Indeed, in several states, parental notification of treatment after the fact is required in instances of pregnancy and venereal disease. Such a situation obtains in Hawaii and Nebraska, although in practice this second step is not always pursued. In yet other laws, physicians are specifically exempted from liability if they notify parents without the minor's concurrence out of a belief that this is still in the minor's best interests. Only in California is the physician enjoined from notifying parents without some sort of indication that the minor agrees with this step, and this applies only to those over 15 years of age who are not living at home.

Insofar as possible, we firmly advocate a position that encourages mature adolescents to be responsible for their own medical affairs, and also respects the fact that they often have both the need for and right to private and confidential health care. But certainly there will be times when parents simply must be informed: when the minor is genuinely in danger of losing his life; when major surgical procedures must be undertaken that pose more than usual risks or will irreparably alter the patient's biological integrity (not including abortions); and/or when the minor is not deemed sufficiently mature as to be able to give a truly informed consent. Under such circumstances we consider that parents' need to know justifiably takes precedence over a minor's right to privacy and confidentiality.

WHO PAYS?

If a minor is deemed capable of consenting to his own health care, the question of who pays is an obvious corollary. While this consideration does not enter into pragmatic, ethical, and legal deliberations about an adolescent's rights and needs, it does raise a most practical point.

Answers are more easily found in relation to less costly ambulatory care. In an office or clinic, a minor may indeed be able to pay his own way if given enough time. When this is not possible, the patient may be referred to low-cost or free facilities; while others will be carried as a debit on the doctor's books, as is frequently done for indigent patients of any age. In other instances, advance arrangements can be made with parents whereby they will pay for their offspring's care but respect its confidential nature, paralleling the usual agreement for minors receiving psychiatric care. One may also hope that health insurers will come to look at this matter and make some sort of provisions for minors who are eligible for confidential health care on their own consent.

But hospitalization poses quite a different problem by virtue of the enormous costs involved. The only presently available alternatives are for minors to call upon their parents' third-party payer (and risk parental notification of this fact); for minors to attempt to seek affirmation of both an indigent and emancipated status in order to obtain Medicaid on their own; or for the hospital to accept the cost of such care as a loss. If a patient's privacy is indeed to be preserved and he cannot qualify for insurance on his own, then the only viable option will be the last alternative, and hospitals will simply have to deal with this fact. Fortunately, it is most unlikely that this problem would come up very often in a given year and such debits should comprise only a tiny fraction of the whole.

MINORS AND "CO-CONSENT"

General Health Care. Up to this point we have dealt with those situations wherein minors may consent to health care on their own in lieu of the parents. But, when parental consent has been obtained and a minor's privacy is not at issue, we wonder just how many hospitals give any thought to obtaining the patient's consent as well. We suspect that they are few indeed. However, we believe that this step is essential and basic to sound and responsive adolescent health care. If one accepts our position that most teen-agers should be involved in making decisions about their own medical affairs, and that the best conditions obtain when the patient functions as a knowledgeable and willing collaborator, then seeking the adolescent's consent to his admission and related procedures, in addition to that of the parents, is fundamental.

Certainly there will be exceptions, such as when the minor is so young that he is unable to give a volitional and informed consent. Also included here are instances involving a potentially fatal disease where it would be wise to keep this diagnosis from the patient—at least for the time being. One can also conceive of situations where the patient is so seriously emotionally or mentally handicapped that he is unable to consent in any meaningful terms. But these are all relatively rare circumstances and it has been our proposition throughout that the vast majority of adolescents not only have the capacity to understand what is going on, but also the need. It is but a short step from this position to consider that the patient's formal consent is an integral part of this process.

From another perspective, there is also a firm indication deriving from case law (e.g., those recent decisions relating to abortions as previously reviewed) that parents cannot enforce a treatment that might be in violation of the youth's own rights or deprive him of determining his own best interests. Parental consent is not absolute, as we have already seen. In light of the growing body of law according minors rights of their own, obtaining a mature minor's consent in addition to that of his parents may be a wise legal precaution.

Research.   The matters discussed above in relation to general medical care are no less applicable to the question of informed consent by minors who are to be subjects of clinical research. At present, there are no definitive guidelines or laws pertinent to this particular matter, although the U.S. Department of Health, Education, and Welfare has proposed regulations for federally funded human investigation that include a provision requiring the consent of minors who are 7 years or more. Certainly, 7-year-olds, with their still limited and concrete thought processes, would be hard put to give any kind of a valid consent that could be considered truly informed. But those who have entered their teen years are generally quite competent in this regard. And, once again, we urge that the consent of adolescents be obtained in all instances of clinical research, except in those same sets of circumstances that would advise against this step for general medical care.

CONFIDENTIALITY IN THE HEALTH CARE RECORD

Confidentiality in the health care record is another often overlooked issue. Yet the consequences of releasing such data to others may have a wide range of unforeseen consequences. This becomes even more critical in the case of adolescents from the perspective of both their as yet unknown futures and present confidential interests.

Health care professionals are generally aware that what they record in the chart remains there in perpetuity. But they may not know that a wide range of persons outside the immediate health care axis may also become privy to even the most personal data. There exists, today, a wide range of data banks that recover and record various pieces of health information without the patient's knowledge, much less with his or her consent. The most significant of these for our interests is the Medical Information Bureau. The computers of MIB contain virtually every diagnosis that has ever been submitted in support of a health insurance claim from member firms. It is estimated that dossiers on some twelve million persons are contained therein, and each can be obtained at will by any one of more than seven hundred participating life and health insurance companies for but a nominal fee. It is true that any citizen now has the right to ask to see his own MIB file and to seek correction or expungement of that which may be erroneous or no longer relevant. But it is doubtful that many patients are even aware of its existence, much less how to gain access thereto. (The MIB is located in Greenwich, Connecticut.)

Until but recently declared an unconstitutional invasion of personal privacy, New York State required that a duplicate of every prescription written for narcotic, barbiturate, and stimulant drugs be submitted to a central office. These data were then entered into a computer in order to identify people who were abusing these agents through multiple licit sources. In another instance, Maryland requires the reporting of sufficient information about patients undergoing abortions so that they can be identified without too much difficulty, even though their names and specific addresses are not involved. This is ostensibly for solely epidemological and demographic purposes, but the potential for abuse exists. A last example rests in regional registries wherein the names of persons receiving any of a variety of services may be entered for purposes of coordination. One such registry in the northeast sector of the United States lists when and where patients have been hospitalized for psychiatric care. Suffice it to say that a multitude of medical "facts" about each one of us who has ever been a patient undoubtedly rests in one or more computers, completely unbeknown to us; and the controls on protecting the confidentiality of such information or the uses to which it may be put are certainly open to question.

As far as the adolescent is concerned, health care professionals must not only be aware of the possible implications for the present if various pieces of information about the minor's health make their way out into the open, but also what these may mean for his future schooling, employment, insurability, and the like. Moreover, the specific confidential interests between an adolescent and his parent also need to be taken into account. Thus within the health care record there may be facts that the youth wishes reserved from his family (such as might pertain to sexual practices) and the reciprocal may be no less true (a history of parental discord or impending divorce). Each will have his own set of vested privacy concerns, and data release must protectively respond.

In making entries into the record and forwarding information on to others, we must be acutely aware of all possible ramifications that this may have and take particular care in both what data we record and the words we use. The responsibility in this matter is great. Even when the patient has given consent for release this can hardly be considered informed. For the patient rarely ever gets to see his own record, has little knowledge of what it contains, and has no concept of what will be passed on. Moreover, when the situation involves a minor, parents are the ones generally asked to consent; and the adolescent will have no opportunity to protect his interests at all.

RECOMMENDATIONS

Nothing can be more confusing and frustrating than the problem posed by an adolescent seeking medical care on his own consent or wishing a health need to be kept confidential. Unless he is clearly emancipated or specific statutes cover the case at hand, few professionals know what to do. Doctors, nurses, or even administrative duty officers cannot be expected to be fully aware of all legally permissible alternatives in relation to minors' consent. But deciding on what course of action to take is often an urgent matter and cannot always wait until the advice of counsel can be sought. We have repeatedly encountered instances where confusion and chaos reigned, or a minor was unwarrantedly deprived of what was clearly his right simply because of the absence of readily available hospital guidelines. Thus, well-conceived policies and procedures are essential.

We strongly urge that hospitals establish a standing committee to establish these policies and procedures; to institute mechanisms for policy review and updating; and to be available for prompt consultation in time of need. We further suggest that this committee not only be composed of administrators and hospital counsel, but also nurses and physicians familiar with adolescent health needs and care delivery, plus a lawyer-advocate to stand on the patient's side. This committee may also wish to include parent and youth representatives.

Hospital Procedures and Policies

1. Existing hospital policies on when and under what circumstances minors may consent to their own health care or be treated without parental consent as an emergency need to be reviewed and updated. Review should take into consideration recent state statutes, relevant case law, the emerging mature minor rule, new directions in minors' rights, expanding definitions of emancipation, and broadening concepts of what constitutes emergency care. When the law, in all its ramifications, still remains unclear, a ruling should be sought from the state's attorney general.

2. Specific policy statements should be developed on defining when minors may consent to their own health care in general and in relation to the following specific medical conditions: veneral disease, contraceptive services, pregnancy detection, prenatal treatment, abortion, sterilization, drug and alcohol abuse, and psychiatric care. Definitions of emancipation for the purposes of medical care and what constitutes an emergency should be established. Policies also will need to be drawn up on what rights minors will be accorded in respecting and maintaining their confidences; and on what exceptions to these rules will obtain (that is, when and under what circumstances parental notification and/or consent shall be permissible or even mandatory).

3. The procedures to be followed in verifying the minor's eligibility to consent to his own health care should also be well defined. What should be written in the chart? Are witnesses or a concurring opinion required and who is eligible to perform these functions? What administrative approval is necessary and who is authorized to give this? What steps are to be followed when the decision as to a minor's eligibility is unclear?

4.   If a minor seeking care on his own consent is not deemed eligible and an emergency does not exist, policies are needed as to whether he may or may not be seen on his own and in private in order to establish the nature of his need and whether he can or cannot at least be counseled on the matter at hand.

5.   When parents cannot accompany a minor who is not eligible to consent to his own care, procedures should be developed for obtaining a valid parental consent, without undue penalty to either youth or parents, through the use of the telephone and/or appropriate consent forms (we consider the requirement of a notarized parental signature to be undue penalty and a regular witness to this act should suffice).

6.   Minors of 12 years or more should consent to their admission, to surgery, to other procedures requiring special consent, and to their participation in clinical research in addition to that of their parents. This should be in as informed a manner as possible consonant with their particular level of maturity. Currently used forms in these matters should be revised accordingly. Exceptions to this general policy will exist and should be defined.

7.   All the preceding policies and procedures should be collated into a single written document and be made readily available to the emergency room, all relevant wards, and the administrative duty officer. Further, a member of the previously recommended hospital committee on consent and confidentiality should be on call for consultation when any questions arise.

Confidentiality and the Health Care Record

1.   An appropriate hospital committee should examine the special interests of minors in this matter and develop policies and procedures both in regard to the minors' and the parents' special confidences one from the other, and in consideration of possible long-range implications of information release.

2.   Consideration should also be given to the concept of the dual record, consisting of a temporary working record and a permanent health care record suitable for release. Data contained in the former are totally restricted and cannot be released, but they must ultimately either be expunged or transferred into the latter.

3.   Minors of 12 years and over as well as their parents should consent to release of health information; and mechanisms need to be established to insure that the consent of both is truly informed and that they know precisely what will be released and to whom. They should also be informed about possibilities

for data storage in computer banks and their rights to review and seek expungement of erroneous material.

Criteria for Applying the Mature Minor Rule

1. We note again that, to our knowledge, no physician has yet been found liable for damages for treating a minor of 16 years or more on his or her own consent for any matter. Thus the arrival of the sixteenth birthday can be seen as a possible determinant of maturity in and of itself.

2. The following points have been offered by the Committee on Youth of the American Academy of Pediatrics as factors to be considered (singly or severally) in assessing whether a minor living at home and not employed is or is not sufficiently mature to consent to his own health care (*Pediatrics* 54:481, 1974). Primarily giving direction in office or out-patient care, with modification they also have relevance for hospitalized youth.

a. The minor makes most of his own decisions about the conduct of his daily affairs.
b. He enjoys substantial independence in his comings and goings from home and moves about easily on his own.
c. Even though supported by parents in major matters, he earns his personal expense money and/or manages most of his day-to-day financial affairs.
d. He has initiated his own medical contact, has come by himself, is able to state his needs, and seems motivated and able to follow through with recommendations on his own.
e. He appears to understand both the risks and benefits of proposed procedures and treatments and thereby is able to give an informed consent.
f. He is unable to communicate readily with his parents about his thoughts and concerns (over the matter at hand—authors' addition).

3. Such guidelines should not, however, be applicable to those minors who are in *serious* risk of life or limb. And parental consent (or at least notification) should be required under these circumstances.

Criteria for Emancipation

1. Each of the following would be widely held as emancipating in and of itself for purposes of a minor's consent to any and all health care, even if not specifically stipulated by law.

a. Age 18 years or more
b. Married
c. A parent (also qualifies these minors to consent to the health care of their child)
d. Living away from home with parental approval, employed and self-supporting

e.   Living at home, but working and contributing at least half of his own support
f.   A member of the armed forces

2.   The following would probably qualify as emancipated, but with somewhat less legal clarity than for the above.

a.   A minor of any age living away from home, making the majority of his own decisions, and managing his own financial affairs; without regard to the status of parental concurrence, the length of separation, or the source of support.
b.   Minor females of any age in relation to pregnancy: that is, prevention, diagnosis, treatment, or termination. (Cf. discussion of pertinent case law, particularly abortions; also note that no physician has, to our knowledge, ever been found liable for damages for providing contraceptive services to a minor of any age.)

Added Legal Protection

Added legal protection in making a judgment of maturity or emancipation for the purposes of consent (in the absence of specific statutory authorization) and in verifying that an informed consent was obtained *may* be provided as follows:

1.   Clearly noting in writing in the patient's chart that the minor was deemed sufficiently mature (or emancipated) as to be eligible to consent to his own health care. This should include the specific evidential items upon which this decision was made.
2.   A written statement in the chart stipulating the specific benefits and risks of the proposed treatment that the patient was advised of and his apparent understanding of these facts. The patient should also sign this statement.
3.   Securing the concurring and written opinion of a second physician that the patient was deemed sufficiently mature (or emancipated) as to be capable of giving an informed consent.
4.   Having an objective "auditor witness" sit in on the discussion of treatment risks and benefits, confirming that an informed consent was obtained, and noting this fact in the chart. This note should also include the name, address, and signature of the "auditor witness."

We recommend that the first and second steps above always be carried out. But, in following items three and four, the possible deleterious effects that introducing a third party might have on the patient's trust and willingness to confide will need to be carefully weighed against the legal protection that this might afford to the physician.

CONCLUSION

In ending this chapter, and indeed this book, we suggest that current legal trends in resolving the dilemma of consent and confidentiality in relation to minor youths reflect the basic philosophy of adolescent health care. For these directions affirm that teen-agers are indeed individuals with their own right to privacy and entitled to exercise it in increasing measure by virtue of a graduating ability to give an informed consent. Recent advances in case and statutory law support this concept and are now rapidly invalidating the old interpretations of common law that long held adolescents to be wholly subject to parental decisions made on their behalf. The adolescent is a person with clear vested interests in all aspects of his medical care and, in his evolving maturity, will come to have more and more private matters of his own. The law in all its present ramifications is becoming increasingly responsive to the minor's emerging, but not quite finished, adulthood.

NOTE: Just as this book was going to press, the United States Supreme Court handed down a particularly significant decision in *Planned Parenthood of Central Missouri* v. *Danforth* (No. 74-1151, 1976). In ruling on the constitutionality of a Missouri law which, in part, required parental consent for abortions in females under 18 years, the Court said: ". . . the State may not impose a blanket provision requiring the consent of a parent or person *in loco parentis* as a condition for abortion of an unmarried minor during the first 12 weeks of her pregnancy. . . . the State does not have the constitutional authority to give a third party an absolute, and possibly arbitrary, veto over the decision of the physician and his patient to terminate the patient's pregnancy. . . . Minors, as well as adults, are protected by the Constitution and possess constitutional rights. . . . Any independent interest the parent may have in the termination of the minor daughter's pregnancy is no more weighty than the right of privacy of the competent minor mature enough to have become pregnant."

This decision does not entirely clear all muddied waters. The construct of the Missouri law and the nature of the appeal was technically such that the Court was required to respond only to the question of parental consent in first trimester abortions and to the extent of the State's regulatory powers thereupon. It did not bar regulations entirely; nor did it address the actual practices of a physician or health facility *per se*.

Nonetheless, the Supreme Court clearly holds State regulations which interfere with a minor's obtaining an abortion to be unconstitutional; acknowledges that minors are no less entitled to privacy than are adults; and firmly supports the mature minor concept. We, ourselves, would further interpret this ruling to have a definite bearing both on second trimester abortions and on a hospital's or physician's abortional practices. We also believe that this decision is even more broadly applicable, offering direction for all health care matters. A general rule can well be drawn which entitles minors to the right to privacy in any patient-physician transaction when mature enough to give an informed consent, particularly when parental consent requirements could be tantamount to depriving them of desired and beneficial care.

selected bibliography

The references cited below are suggested as additional readings for those who wish to pursue particular topics in greater depth. Each entry has been assigned to that chapter for which it has the greatest relevance, but many will have significance for other chapters as well.

Chapter 1. Critical Issues of Normal Adolescence

Blos, P. Character formation in adolescence. *Psychoanal Study Child* 23:245, 1968.

———. The second individuation process of adolescence. *Psychoanal Study Child* 22:162, 1967.

Caplan, H. Some considerations of the body image concept in child development. *Q J Child Behavior* 4:382, 1952.

Deutsch, H. *Selected Problems of Adolescence*. New York: International Universities Press, 1967.

Erikson, E. H. *Childhood and society*. 2d ed. New York: W. W. Norton, 1963.

———. *The challenge of youth*. Garden City, N.Y.: Doubleday, 1965.

Freud, A. Observations on child development. *Psychoanal Study Child* 6:18, 1951.

———. Adolescence. *Psychoanal Study Child* 13:255, 1958.

Group for the Advancement of Psychiatry. *Normal adolescence: its dynamics and impact*. New York: Group for the Advancement of Psychiatry, 1968.

Inhelder, B., and J. Piaget. *The growth of logical thinking from childhood to adolescence*. London: Routledge & Kegan Paul, 1958.

Josselyn, I. M. *The adolescent and his world*. New York: Family Service Association of America, 1952.

Schilder, P. *Image and appearance of the human body*. New York: International Universities Press, 1950.

Schonfeld, W. A. Body image in adolescence: A psychiatric concept for the pediatrician. *Pediatrics* 31:845, 1963.

Tanner, J. M. *Growth at adolescence.* 2d ed. Oxford: Blackwell, 1962.

Winnicott, D. W. *The collected papers: Through pediatrics to psycho-analysis.* London: Tavistock, 1958.

Chapter 2. The Impact of Illness

Cooper, H. Psychological aspects of congenital heart disease. *S Afr Med J* 33:349, 1952.

Boyle, I. R., P. A. di Sant'Agnese, S. Sack, F. Millican, and L. L. Kulczycki. Emotional adjustment of adolescents and young adults with cystic fibrosis. *J Pediatr* 88:318, 1976.

Engel, G. K. Psychogenic pain. *Med Clin North Am* 42:1481, 1958.

————. A unified concept of health and disease. *Perspect Biol Med* 3:459, 1960.

Finley, K. H., S. T. Buse, R. W. Popper, M. P. Honzink, D. S. Collart, and N. Riggs. Intellectual functioning of children with tetralogy of Fallot: Influence of open-heart sugrery and earlier palliative operations. *J Pediatr* 85:318, 1974.

Freeman, R. D. Psychiatric problems in adolescents with cerebral palsy. *Devel Med Child Neurol* 12:64, 1970.

Freud, A. The role of body illness in the mental life of children. *Psychoanal Study Child* 7:69, 1952.

————. Severe, chronic versus minor, acute illness. In *Children in the hospital,* ed. T. Bergman, pp. 135–51. New York: International Universities Press, 1965.

Garson, A., Jr., R. B. Williams, and J. Reckless. Long-term follow-up of patients with tetralogy of Fallot: Physical health and psychopathology. *J Pediatr* 85:429, 1974.

Kann, M. M. R. The concept of cumulative trauma. *Psychoanal Study Child* 18:286, 1963.

Kassebaum, G., and B. Baumann. Dimensions of the sick role in chronic illness. In *Patients, physicians, and illness,* ed. E. G. Jaco, pp. 141–54. New York: Free Press, 1972.

Kaufman, R. V. Body-image changes in physically ill teenagers. *J Am Acad Child Psychiatry* 11:157, 1972.

———— and B. Hersher. Body image changes in teenage diabetics. *Pediatrics* 48:123, 1971.

Kolb, L. C. Disturbances in body image. In *American handbook of psychiatry,* ed. S. Arieti, pp. 749–69. New York: Basic Books, 1959.

Lipowski, Z. J. Psychosocial aspects of disease. *Ann Intern Med* 71:1197, 1969.

Little, S. Psychology of physical illness in adolescents. *Ped Clin North Am* 7:85, 1960.

Meissner, A. L., R. W. Thoreson, and A. J. Butler. Relation of self-concept to impact and obviousness of disability among male and female adolescents. *Percept Motor Skills* 24:1099, 1967.

Partridge, J. W., A. M. Garner, C. W. Thompson, and T. Cherry. Attitudes of adolescents toward diabetes. *Am J Dis Child* 124:226, 1972.

Pless, I. B., and K. J. Roghmann. Chronic illness and its consequences: Observations based on three epidemiologic surveys. *J Pediatr* 79:351, 1971.

Spilken, A. Z., and M. A. Jacobs. Prediction of illness behavior from measures of life crisis, manifest distress and maladaptive coping. *Psychosom Med* 33:251, 1971.

Watson, E. J., and A. M. Johnson. The emotional significance of acquired physical disfigurement in children. *Am J Orthopsychiatry* 28:85, 1958.

Whitehouse, F. A. Problems of the cardiac adolescent. *NY State J Med* 64:1108, 1964.

Willis, J. E. Emotional problems associated with chronic organic illness. In *New dimensions in psychosomatic medicine,* ed. C. W. Wahl, pp. 291–303. Boston: Little, Brown, 1964.

Chapter 3.   The Implications and Course of Hospitalization

Abram, H. S. Psychological aspects of surgery. *Int Psychiatry Clin* 4:vii, 1967.

Bergmann, T., in collaboration with A. Freud. *Children in the hospital.* New York: International Universities Press, 1965.

Bodley, P. O., H. V. R. Jones, and M. D. Mather. Pre-operative anxiety: A qualitative analysis. *J Neurol Neurosurg Psychiatry* 37:230, 1974.

Conway, B. The effect of hospitalization on adolescence. *Adolescence* 6:77, 1971.

Haller, A. J., ed. *The hospitalized child.* Baltimore: Johns Hopkins Press, 1968.

Robinson, L. *Psychological aspects of the care of hospitalized patients.* Philadelphia: F. A. Davis, 1972.

Sargent, D. A. Confinement and ego-regression: Some consequences of enforced passivity. *Psychiatry Med* 5, 1974.

Swanson, D. W. Clinical psychiatric problems associated with general surgery. *Int Psychiatry Clin* 4:58, 1967.

Vernon, D. T. A., J. M. Foley, R. R. Sipowicz, and J. L. Schulman. *Psychological responses of children to hospitalization and illness.* Springfield, Ill.: Charles C. Thomas, 1965.

Chapter 4.   Coping with Stress

Chodoff, P. Adjustment to disability. *J Chronic Dis* 9:653, 1959.

————, S. B. Friedman, and D. A. Hamburg. Stress defenses and coping behavior: Observations in parents of children with malignant disease. *Am J Psychiatry* 121:743, 1964.

Hamburg, D. A., and J. E. Adams. A perspective on coping behaviors. *Arch Gen Psychiatry* 17:277, 1967.

Hofmann, A. D. The impact of illness in adolescence and coping behavior. *Acta Pediatr Scand* Sup. no. 256, pp. 29–33, 1975.

Myers, B. A., S. B. Friedman, and I. B. Weinger. Coping with a chronic disability. *Am J Dis Child* 120:175, 1970.

Visotsky, W. M. Coping behavior under extreme stress. *Arch Gen Psychiatry* 5:423, 1961.

Weinstein, E. A., and R. L. Kahn. *Denial of illness.* Springfield, Ill.: Charles C. Thomas, 1955.

Chapter 5.   Ward Staff Interactions among Themselves, Patients, and Parents

Artiss, K. L., and A. S. Levine. Doctor-patient relations in severe illness. *N Engl J Med* 288:1210, 1973.

Beckhard, R. *Organization development: Strategies and models.* Reading, Mass.: Addison-Wesley, 1969.

Fuzzard, M. B. Acceptance of authoritarianism in the nurse by the hospitalized teen-ager. *Nurs Res* 18:426, 1969.

Kaplan DeNour, A., and J. W. Czackes. Emotional problems and reactions of the medical team in a chronic hemodialysis unit. *Lancet* 2:987, 1968.

Kessler, K., and T. Weiss. Ward-staff problems with abortions. *Psychiatry Med* 5, 1974.

Raimbault, G., O. Cachin, J. M. Limal, C. Eliacheff, and R. Rappaport. Aspects of communication between patients and doctors: An analysis of the discourse in medical interviews. *Pediatrics* 55:401, 1975.

Revens, R. W. *Standards for morale: Cause and effect in hospitals*. London: Oxford University Press, 1964.

Rothenberg, M. B. Reactions of those who treat children with cancer. *Pediatrics* 40:507, 1967.

Chapter 6. The Hospital Setting

Bach, W. G. Teen-aged patients. *Hospitals* 44:51, 1970.

Glaser, H., G. Coffin, and P. Christie. *Changing hospital environments for children*. Cambridge, Mass.: Harvard University Press, 1973.

Rigg, C. A., and R. C. Fisher. Some comments on current hospital medical services for adolescents. *Am J Dis Child* 120:193, 1970.

Schowalter, J. E. and W. R. Anyan. Experience on an adolescent in-patient division. *Am J Dis Child* 125:212, 1973.

———— and R. D. Lord. Admission to an adolescent ward. *Pediatrics* 46:1009, 1970.

Society for Adolescent Medicine, Committee on Inpatient Care. Characteristics of an inpatient unit for adolescents. *Clin Pediatr* 12:17, 1973.

Chapter 7. Optimal Staff Roles and Relationships

Bates, B. Doctor and nurse: Changing roles and relations. *N Engl J Med* 283:129, 1970.

Beckhard, R. Organizational issues in the team delivery of comprehensive health care. *Milbank Fund Quarterly* (July 1972), pp. 287–316.

Bibring, G. E. Psychiatry and medical practice in a general hospital. *N Engl J Med* 254:366, 1956.

Fineman, A. D. The utilization of child psychiatry on a surgical service. *Am J Surg* 95:64, 1958.

Freud, A. Pediatricians' questions answered. In *Psychosomatic aspects of paediatrics,* ed. R. C. MacKeith and J. Sandler. New York: Pergamon, 1961.

Meyer, B. C. Some considerations of the doctor-patient relationship in the practice of surgery. *Int Psychiatry Clin* 4:17, 1967.

Rothenberg, M. B. Child psychiatry-pediatrics liaison: A history and commentary. *J Am Acad Child Psychiatry* 7:492, 1968.

Rubin, I. M., and R. Beckhard. Factors influencing the effectiveness of health teams. *Milbank Fund Quarterly* (July 1972), pp. 317–335.

Winnicott, D. W. *Therapeutic consultations in child psychiatry.* London: Hogarth, 1971.

Chapter 8.   Patient Care from Admission to Discharge

Daniel, W. A. *The adolescent patient.* St. Louis: C. V. Mosby, 1970.

Gallagher, J. R., F. P. Heald, and D. C. Garell, eds. *Medical care of the adolescent.* 3d ed. New York: Appleton-Century-Crofts, 1975.

Hofmann, A. D., and R. D. Becker. Psychotherapeutic approaches to the physically ill adolescent. *Int J Child Psychotherapy* 2:492, 1973.

Oremland, M. E., and J. Oremland. *The effects of hospitalization on children: Models for their care.* Springfield, Ill.: Charles C. Thomas, 1973.

Thompson, H. Assisting parents with post-hospitalization plans. *J Amer Hosp Assoc* 4:43, 1973.

Chapter 9.   Common Behavioral Problems

Gerstman, J. Psychological and phenomenological aspects of disorders of the body-image. *J Nerv Ment Dis* 126:499, 1958.

Hofmann, A. D. Adolescents in distress: Suicide and out-of-control behaviors. *Med Clin North Am* 59:1429, 1975.

Joffe, W. G., and J. Sandler. Notes on pain, depression, and individuation. *Psychoanal Study Child* 20:394, 1965.

Kalogerakis, M., ed. *The emotionally troubled youth and the family physician.* Springfield, Ill.: Charles C. Thomas, 1973.

Lorand, S. Adolescent depression. *Int J. Psychoanal* 48:53, 1967.

Scharl, A. E. Regression and restitution in object loss. *Psychoanal Study Child* 16:471, 1961.

Schmale, A. Relationship of preparation and depression to disease. *Psychosom Med* 20:259, 1958.

Weiner, I. *Psychological disturbance in adolescence.* New York: Wiley-Interscience, 1970.

Wise, T. N. Psychiatric management of patients who threaten to sign out against medical advice. *Psychiatry Med* 5, 1974.

Chapter 10.   Particularly Difficult Situations and Stressful Procedures

Abram, H. S. Adaptation to open-heart surgery: A psychiatric study of response to the threat of death. *Am J Psychiatry* 122:659, 1965.

Abrams, R. D. The patient with cancer: His changing pattern of communication. *N Engl J Med* 274:317, 1966.

Aisenberg, R. B., P. Wolff, A. Rosenthal, and A. S. Nadas. Psychological impact of cardiac catheterization. *Pediatrics* 51:1051, 1973.

Andreasen, N. J. C., R. Noyes, C. E. Hartford, G. Brodland, and S. Proctor. Management of emotional reactions in seriously burned adults. *N Engl J Med* 286:65, 1972.

Bernstein, D. M. After transplantation: The child's emotional reaction. *Am J Psychiatry* 127:1189, 1971.

Castelnuovo-Tedesco, P. Introduction: Psychiatric aspects of organ transplantation. *Semin Psychiatry* 3, 1971.

Cohen, S., A. E. Silverman, and B. M. Shmavonian. Psychological studies in altered sensory environments. *J Psychosom Res* 6:259, 1962.

Danilowicz, D. A., and H. P. Gabriel. Post-operative reactions in children: "Normal" and "abnormal" responses following cardiac surgery. *Am J Psychiatry* 128:185, 1971.

———. Post-cardiotomy psychosis in non-English-speaking patients. *Psychiatry Med* 2:314, 1971.

Egerton, N., and J. H. Kay. Psychological disturbances associated with open-heart surgery. *Br J. Psychiatry* 110:433, 1964.

Friedman, E. A., N. J. Goodwin, and L. Cahudhry. Psychosocial adjustment to maintenance hemodialysis. Part I. *NY State J Med* 70:629, 1970.

Golden, J. S., and A. Nahum. Emotional reactions to mutilating surgery. *New Dimensions in Psychosomat Med* 17:201, 1964.

Heller, S. S., K. A. Frank, J. R. Malm, F. O. Bowman, P. D. Harris, M. H. Charlton, and D. S. Kornfeld. Psychiatric complications of open-heart surgery: A re-examination. *N Engl J Med* 283:1015, 1970.

Holland, J., J. M. Sgroi, S. J. Marwit, and N. Solkoff. The ICU syndrome: Fact or fancy? *Psychiatry Med* 4:241, 1973.

Kemph, J. P. Psychotherapy with patients receiving kidney transplants. *Am J Psychiatry* 124:623, 1967.

King, M. Evaluation and treatment of suicide-prone youth. *Mental Hygiene* 55:344, 1971.

Kohlberg, I. J., and M. D. Rothenberg. Comprehensive care following multiple life-threatening injuries: Treatment of an adolescent boy. *Am J Dis Child* 119:449, 1970.

Kornfeld, D. A., S. Zimberg, and J. R. Malm. Psychiatric complications of open-heart surgery. *N Engl J Med* 273:287, 1965.

Korsch, B. M., V. F. Negrete, J. E. Gardner, C. L. Weinstock, A. S. Mercer, C. M. Grushkin, and R. N. Fine. Kidney transplantation in children: Psychosocial follow-up study on child and family. *J Pediatr* 83:399, 1973.

Layne, O. L., Jr., and S. C. Yodofsky. Postoperative psychosis in cardiotomy patients. *N Engl J Med* 284:518, 1971.

Lazarus, H. R., and J. H. Hagens. Prevention of psychosis following open-heart surgery. *Am J Psychiatry* 124:1190, 1968.

Margolis, G. J. Post-operative psychosis on the intensive care unit. *Compr Psychiatry* 8:227, 1967.

Moore, D. C., C. P. Hilton, and G. W. Marten. Psychological problems in the management of adolescents with malignancy. *Clin Pediatr* 8:464, 1969.

Nordan, R., R. Ostendorf, and J. P. Naughton. Return to the land of the living: An approach to the problem of chronic hemodialysis. *Pediatrics* 48:939, 1971.

Richmond, J. B., and H. A. Waisman. Psychological aspects of management of children with malignant disease. *Am J Dis Child* 89:42, 1955.

Seligman, R. A psychiatric classification system for burned children. *Am J Psychiatry* 131:1, 1974.

Stanley, E. J., and J. T. Barter. Adolescent suicidal behavior. *Am J Orthopsychiatry* 40:87, 1970.

Teicher, J. D. A solution to the chronic problem of living: Adolescent attempted suicide. In *Current issues in adolescent psychiatry,* ed. J. C. Schoolar, pp. 129–47. New York: Brunner/Mazel, 1973.

Weinberg, S. Suicidal intent in adolescence: A hypothesis about the role of physical illness. *J Pediatr* 77:579, 1970.

Chapter 11.   Neurological and Orthopedic Handicaps

Anderson, T. P., and T. M. Cole. Sexual counseling of the physically disabled. *Postgrad Med* 58:117, 1975.

Barker, R. H., B. A. Wright, and H. R. Golvick. *Adjustment to physical handicap and illness.* Bulletin no. 55. New York: Social Science Research Council, 1946.

Bax, M., and R. MacKeith. The results of treatment. *Devel Med Child Neurol* 9:2, 1967.

Cruickshank, W. M. The effects of physical disability on personal aspiration. *J Child Behavior* 3:323, 1951.

Easson, W. M. Psychopathological environmental reactions to congenital defects. *J Nerv Ment Dis* 5:453, 1956.

Freeman, R. D. Psychiatric problems in adolescents with cerebral palsy. *Devel Med Child Neurol* 12:64, 1970.

Grayson, A. *Psychiatric aspects of rehabilitation.* Rehabilitation monographs no. 2. New York: New York University Institute of Physical Medicine and Rehabilitation, 1952.

Kennedy, J. M. *Orthopaedic splints and appliances.* London: Baillière-Tindall, 1974.

Kimmel, J. A comparison of children with congenital and acquired orthopedic handicaps on certain personality characteristics. *Dissertation Abstracts* 19:3023, 1959.

McDaniel, J. *Physical disability and human behavior.* Oxford: Pergamon, 1972.

Sheelhase, L. J. and E. Fern. Role of the family in rehabilitation. *Social Casework* 53:544, 1972.

Shotland, L. Social work approaches to the chronically handicapped and their families. *Social Work* 9:4:68, 1964.

Weiss, A. J., and M. D. Diamond. Psychologic adjustment of patients with myelopathy. *Arch Phys Med Rehab* 47:72, 1966.

————. Sexual adjustment, identification and attitudes of patients with myelopathy. *Arch Phys Med Rehab* 47:245, 1966.

Wilson, W. P., and S. N. Blaine. Psychiatric considerations of certain neurological diseases treated neuro-surgically. *Int Psychiat Clin* 4:2:189, 1967.

Chapter 12. The Dying Adolescent

Abrams, R. D. The patient with cancer: His changing pattern of communication. *N Engl J Med* 274:317, 1966.

Beard, B. H. Fear of death and fear of life. *Arch Gen Psychiatry* 21:373, 1969.

Bowlby, J. Childhood mourning and its implications for psychiatry. *Am J Psychiatry* 118:481, 1961.

Easson, W. M. *The dying child: The management of the child or adolescent who is dying.* Springfild, Ill.: Charles C. Thomas, 1970.

Friedman, S. B., P. Chodoff, J. W. Mason, and D. A. Hamburg. Behavioral observations in parents anticipating the death of a child. *Pediatrics* 32:610, 1963.

Group for the Advancement of Psychiatry. *Death and dying: Attitudes of patient and doctor.* New York: Group for the Advancement of Psychiatry, 1968.

Ingles, T. Death on a ward. *Nursing Outlook* 12:28, 1965.

Kübler-Ross, E. *On death and dying.* New York: Macmillan, 1970.

Morrissey, J. R. A note on interviews with children facing imminent death. *Social Casework* 44:343, 1963.

McIntire, M. S., C. B. Angle, and L. S. Struempler. The concept of death in midwestern children and youth. *Am J Dis Child* 122:527, 1972.

Quint, J. C. Obstacles to helping the dying. *Am J Nursing* 66:1568, 1966.

Reich, R., and H. B. Feinberg. The fatally ill adolescent. In *Adolescent psychiatry,* ed. S. C. Feinstein and P. Giovacchini, vol. 3, pp. 75–85. New York: Basic Books, 1974.

Roseman, L., and L. Sechrest. Attitudes of registered nurses toward death in a general hospital. *Psychiatry Med* 4:411, 1973.

Schoenberger, B., A. Carr, D. Peretz, and A. H. Kutscher, eds. *Loss and grief: Psychological management in medical practice.* New York: Columbia University Press, 1970.

Solnit, A. J. The dying child. *Neurology* 7:693, 1965.

Chapter 13. Consent and Confidentiality

American Academy of Pediatrics, Committee on Youth. The implications of minor's consent legislation for adolescent health care: A commentary. *Pediatrics* 54:481, 1974.

American Psychiatric Association. *Confidentiality: A report of the 1974 conference on confidentiality of health care records.* Washington: American Psychiatric Association, 1975.

Chayet, N. I. *Legal implications of emergency care.* New York: Appleton-Century-Crofts, 1969.

Curran, W. J., and H. K. Beecher. Experimentation in children. *J AMA* 210:77, 1969.

Family Planning/Population Reporter. (This excellent quarterly journal reviews and updates state laws and policies influencing family planning, including minors' consent laws. It is available by subscription—currently $18/yr.—from Allan Guttmacher Institute Publications, 1666 K St. NW, Washington, D.C. 20006.)

Hofmann, A. D. Confidentiality and the health care records of children and youth. *Psychiatric Opinion* 12:20, 1975.

————. Is confidentiality in health care records a pediatric concern? *Pediatrics* 57:170, 1976.

———— and H. F. Pilpel. The legal rights of minors. *Ped Clin North Am* 20:989, 1973.

National Center for Family Planning Services. *Family planning, contraception, and voluntary sterilization: An analysis of laws and policies in the United States (each state and jurisdiction as of September 1971).* DHEW pub. no. (HSA) 74-16001. Washington: Government Printing Office, 1974.

Paul, E. W., H. F. Pilpel, and N. W. Wechsler. Pregnancy, teenagers, and the law, 1974. *Family Planning Perspectives* 6:142, 1974.

Schwartz, A. H. Children's concepts of research hospitalization. *N Engl J Med* 287:589, 1972.

The rights of children. Part I. *Harvard Educational Review* vol. 43, no. 4 (1973).

The rights of children. Part II. *Harvard Educational Review* vol. 44, no. 1 (1974).

Zuckerman, R. J. Abortion and contraception: A minor's constitutional right to privacy. *Family Planning/Population Reporter* 4:114, 1975.

index

A

Abortion, 102, 183, 215, 220, 232
Accidents, 175–178
Acne, 130, 132
Acting out, 62–64, 158–159
Acute illness, 137–139
Acute reaction phase, 42–44, 45
Admission, 39–41, 122–123
    elective, 134–135
    repeated, 171–172
Adolescence
    cultural modifiers, 17
    early, 14–15
    emancipation, 4, 5, 9–10, 15, 20,
        217–218, 230–231
    functional identity, 12–13
    intellectual development, 10–12
    late, 16–17
    mid-, 15–16
    puberty, 4, 5–8, 130–132
    role definition, 10–13
    sexual identity, 12, 17, 27, 168–169
    stages of, 13–17
Adolescent medicine specialist, 99,
        108–109, 115, 117
Alienation, 4
Amputation, 39, 173–175
Anger, 80–82
Announcement of hospitalization, 37–39
Anorexia nervosa, 31, 173
Anticipation phase, 42
Anxiety: see Stress, coping with
Asthma, 23, 31
Autonomy, 20–21
Avoidance, 79, 199

B

Bathroom facilities, 94, 97
Behavioral problems, 149–169
    acting out, 158–159
    agitated states, 152
    borderline psychosis, 155
    chronic illness, 142
    depression and withdrawal, 154,
        165–166
    environmental involvement, 164–165
    guilt, 153
    high-risk groups, 151–153
    impulse disorders, 156
    limit setting, 163–164
    management principles, 159–167
    organically impaired mental functions,
        154–155
    panic, 159, 166–167
    permanent handicaps and mutilations,
        153
    preexisting emotional problems,
        151–152
    provocative and manipulative behaviors,
        156–158
    psychiatric liaison, 167
    sexually provocative behaviors, 167–169
    staff-patient relationship, 162–163
    ventilation, 161–162
Blos, P., 9
Borderline psychosis, 155

C

Causality of illness, 30–31
Cerebral palsy, 188, 191–192
Chronic illness, 21–24, 139–142
    acute exacerbations, 139–140
    behavioral problems, 142
    coordination of care, 141–142
    deterioration, 141
    diagnostic evaluation, 140
    hospitalization and, 44–46
    recurrent hospitalization for, 171–173
    special therapies, 140–141
Clergy, 73, 114
Comatose patient, 200–201
Communication gaps, 87–88
Compensation, 59–60, 62

Confidentiality, 226–227, 229–230
Consent, 211–232
case law, 215–217
statutory law, 218–222
Supreme Court, 215, 232
Convalescence, 142–146
early, 142–143
late, 145–146
mid- 143–145
Coping mechanisms: *see* Stress, coping with
Countertransference, 198
Crushes, 15
Cultural modifiers of adolescence, 17

D

Dating, 15, 16, 128
Death: *see* Dying adolescent
Defense mechanisms: *see* Stress, coping with
Denial, 55–56, 77, 78–79, 174–175
Depression, 145, 154, 165–166
Diabetics, 19, 23
Diagnostic evaluation, 140
Dialysis, 178–179, 210
Diet, 94–95, 98
Disfigurements, 28–29, 39, 153, 173–175
Displacement, 60–62
Doctors, 68–71, 99, 107–109, 115–117
Drug abuse, 4
Duodenal ulcer, 31
Dying adolescent, 24, 196–210
acute death, 200–201
dialysis, 210
at home, 209–210
management, 201–208
parents and, 197–198, 206, 208, 209
staff and, 198–199, 202–208
in teaching hospital, 208–209
treatment controversies, 209
ward structure, 202–203

E

Early adolescence, 14–15
Early convalescence, 142–143
Education, 72, 95, 98, 113–114, 144
Emancipation, 4, 5, 9–10, 15, 20, 217–218, 230–231
Emergency care, consent and, 220–222
Emotionally disturbed adolescents, hospitalization and, 48–50
Epilepsy, 23
Erikson, E. H., 9

F

Family Educational Rights and Privacy Act of 1975, 212–213
Fantasy life, 12, 19, 26, 35
Freud, Anna, xi–xiii, 9
Frustration, 80–82
Functional identity, 12–13

G

Greenspan, Leon, 188–195
Group therapy, 161–162
Growth at Adolescence (Tanner), 6
Guilt, 30–31, 50, 153, 199
Gynecological patient, 101–102

H

Heart disease, 23
Hersher, B., 19
Hodgkin's disease, 23
Hospital setting, 91–103, 121–122
bathroom facilities, 94, 97
education, 95, 98
general principles, 92–95
ideal, 95–99
intensive care unit, 100
intermediate care unit, 100–101
interviewing and counseling rooms, 97
isolation, 101
nursing station, 97
obstetrical and gynecological patient, 101–102
patients' rooms, 92, 96–97
recreation room, 92–93, 97–98
treatment room, 97
Hospitalization, 33–53; *see also* Hospital setting; Patient care; Staff
acute reaction phase, 42–44, 45
admission, 39–41
announcement of, 37–39
anticipation phase, 42
chronic illness, 44–46